Fearless

My Journey That Healed Breast Cancer – *and my life*, Through Faith, Food and Fun.

Venus DeMarco

with

Lisa Smith

Cover illustration by April Bensch, Myrtle Beach, SC
Cover Design by Jason K Wheeler, Pawley's Island, SC

ASPENHILL Publishing Group
1520 Senate Street
Suite 67
Columbia, SC 29201
803 446 9361
http://www.aspenhillpublishing.co
(the web address ends in .co rather than .com)

Printed in the United States of America by Fidelity Printing
www.FidelityPrinting.com
Second Edition: January 2016
10 9 8 7 6 5 4 3 2

The publisher is not responsible for websites (or their content) not owned by the publisher.

ISBN: 978-0-9860452-7-1

Foreword

If you have this book in your hand, there is a reason. God loves and cares about you so much and wants you to know that you are not walking through this life alone. He created our bodies and, as Venus so clearly shows us in this book, He can also heal them.

If you are looking for ways to heal your body of cancer or, if you just want to learn more ways to prevent it, this book is for you. Probably what I like the best about it - and Venus herself, is how completely honest she is.

None of us have all of the answers. In fact, given the statistics on cancer, none of us may have any of the answers. That's why she calls it her 'journey'. Everyone who gets a diagnosis of cancer begins a journey. Venus shows how important it is to take a personal interest in our own and how to not just let the doctors take you anywhere they want.

While chemo, radiation and surgeries are their 'go to' strategies, Venus stood up and said 'No!' She showed that a woman doesn't have to lose her breasts and her hair to save her life. Not every woman has the strength – or faith, of Venus and that's why she wrote this book. She wants to share with you what she has learned. She also wants to tell you how God gave her the courage to push through the fear and walk by faith, not by sight.

More than anything, Venus wants you to live! She truly cares about each individual she meets – or even hears about, with such compassion and empathy that you'd think you were her very own family. This book will give you courage and bring healing to your life - not because of Venus but, rather instead, because of the One who guided her. So, enjoy each page as she shows you how – through faith, food and fun, to walk on the path of your own journey of complete healing.

John S Pruett,
The Amorvita Foundation

Introduction

Let me ask you: is it the fear or the disease?

As serious as the subject of cancer is, this book will take you from laughter to tears and will leave you with your eyes wide open to the truth about cancer and healing. Come along with me as I travel through the Disneyland of cancer treatment centers, to the Redneck Riviera and over the border of Mexico to discover the truth about healing. The road I took would prove to be difficult at times. As a matter of fact, I ran into Goliath along the way and had to gather up enough courage to stand face to face with him.

But, it was in the midst of my search for answers - with fear breathing down my neck, that blind faith taught me to say it was really over from the moment I was diagnosed - I just didn't realize it. Healing is a gift from God and I have found that practicing good nutrition is a wonderful path that allows me to live a long, healthy, and productive life. My hope is that my story will inspire not only women but men also to not 'become' their disease and, if ever diagnosed with cancer, to give them the chance to have peace of mind much sooner than I did. Learning the truth truly *does* set you free!

I am not a celebrity or a wealthy individual. I am a single, self-employed woman in my 50's and in the same economic situation shared by many others today. Since the diagnosis, I have been speaking to various groups throughout the United States on the topic, "Is it the fear, or is it the disease?" and other topics having to do with the health of our body, mind and spirit. I am also passionate about encouraging those who have decided to take the natural route versus the conventional route.

My website, *www.VenusDeMarco.org*, contains information for those who are seeking knowledge to live a healthier, happier life, including recipes, blogs and even a nutritional supplements store.

Soon after I was diagnosed, I began talking about a book that I was going to write which would take the fear out of individuals' hearts. This is that book and it is for anyone who has breast cancer or, cancer of any kind. It is also for those who simply enjoy an inspirational story.

My prayer is this book will lead to more conversations about the potential for preventing and curing cancer and other diseases through lifestyle changes. And, more than anything that this book helps take the fear out of your heart when it comes to cancer!

Sincerely,

Venus DeMarco

Dedications

Living this journey and writing this book has forever changed my life. I would love to thank God, my Lord Jesus and the comfort of His Holy Spirit along with the following people for all they did in their own special way:

Gayle, for being there from the beginning, always helping me spiritually, emotionally, and even financially. I will never be able to thank you enough. To **Teresa Tapp** for believing in me from the start - even when you didn't really know me. Thank you so much for giving me my first speaking gig to tell my story. You awoke the best in me. Most of all, for your belief in this book. **Lisa**, without you and your ability to sit me down, listen, and record my whole story, I don't know if it would have ever gotten done. Thank you for helping me get this on paper. I will forever be grateful. **Charlotte**, for kicking me in the butt to get this thing started. To my sister **Shaula**, who I love more than anyone in the world. I know this wasn't easy for you especially because - at first, you didn't understand what I was doing. To **Brenda**, **Janelle**, and all the **Ta Ta Sisterhood** - you know who you are - just know I hold all of you close to my heart. **Jan**, **Pilar** and **Cindy**, for calling me every day for at least two years to see how I was doing, encouraging me, and praying for me. God Bless you. **Pilar**, for the many Whole Foods gift cards. **Victor**, for your friendship and love. Even when you were in Afghanistan defending our freedoms, you were right here with me. To my wonderful clients and friends, who took this bumpy road with me and didn't leave. Thank you! To **Doc Cotter** and **Mark Johnson**, thank you for your hospitality and being there for me in the beginning. To my **Aunt Jo** and **Aunt Nancy**, you two wonderful people. **Pam**, thank you for just being you. **Cathy De Marco**, I feel like you are my other sister. **Shelly**, for spending your birthday with me - what a night! And then bringing **Hot Al** and **Sophia** to Austin for Thanksgiving… we are friends for life - that's what you always say!

Last but not least, thank you to my lovable, quirky **Iggy**.

7

Contents

Good Friday

As I wake up to another gorgeous day in Austin, Texas, I glance over to see my handsome dog Iggy asleep in his bed. It's at this very moment - before my feet hit the floor, that I take time to tell God how grateful I am. For the last two years, I have consistently started my day off by thanking Him for healing me and showing me that I am a victor - not a victim. I cannot begin to tell you the depth of strength, courage, wisdom and grace that He has filled my heart with.

Where did all of this start? Flipping through my journal I find the date,

April 10th, 2009 *I hear the words that bring instant fear to so many people: "Venus you have breast cancer." Shockingly enough, it is no surprise to me. You see, this very large mass that is approximately 9 centimeters has*

been there for almost six months. When it was obvious that the mass was abnormal, I asked my sister, who is a personal trainer, if I had pulled a muscle in my breast. She said, "Venus, you know that muscle tissue isn't on top of the breast."

The year and a half prior to that day, I had started doing a wellness program called *T-Tapp*. *T-Tapp* is a method of movement that is a compound muscle workout. This means it uses the full length of the muscle plus supporting muscles at the same time - full fiber muscle activation. It's neurokinetic, meaning it connects your mind to your body. Like the old saying, "Use it or lose it," this exercise keeps the mind youthful. Most important to me though, it's a lymphatic workout meaning that it stimulates lymphatic flow which optimizes the lymph system. This means it moves waste out at a cellular level. The lymphatic system, for those who don't know, takes the trash out of the body. I had enjoyed the work outs so much that, at the time of the diagnosis, I was studying to be a trainer.

At that particular time, I was in Houston participating in a T-Tapp workshop in which we worked out for four straight hours at a time. I felt great even though I was experiencing a terrible time with hot flashes.

I remember waking up at 4 a.m. that night from a rash on my arms. The bumps were white with red dots and covered both of my arms from the shoulder to the middle of my biceps. Strangely the rash didn't itch. I just thought that the workout I had been doing triggered the rash somehow. However, in addition to the rash, I had been experiencing a lot of pain in my right breast whenever I laid on my side or flat on my stomach. So, I knew something wasn't right.

I had always heard that breast cancer wasn't painful and that the lumps were round like marbles or shaped like a hard pea. The mass on my breast was completely opposite of those descriptions. It was long and tubular in appearance and extremely painful at times. That being said, six months is a long period of time to ignore symptoms like mine. It wasn't that I was in denial; I just wasn't quite ready to do anything about it.

The time finally came when I was ready to address the symptoms that were affecting my bodacious Ta Ta's. I scheduled an appointment with a nurse practitioner to get a referral for a mammogram. They quickly determined that something was wrong and rushed me to the ultrasound room. It was right out of one those old prison movies - the good prisoners are released for some recreation while the ones who are in trouble are returned to their cells. It was crystal clear which patients were potential prisoners of breast cancer, that's for sure. There we waited in the ultrasound 'cell' with the blank look of fear on our faces.

After a long and painful ultra sound, the radiologist came into the room and was frantically animated as she told me they had found a very large mass on my breast - like I hadn't noticed. The only good thing she said to me during my appointment was, "Venus, at least there's always hope."

Once she left the room, I mentioned to the ultrasound technician that the radiologist really should consider a career change. With her excessive drama skills, she would be a great kindergarten teacher keeping kids entertained for long periods of time.

As I left the doctor's office that afternoon, I remembered walking out to my car feeling scared and afraid. I was all alone. I sat there crying, not knowing what to do next. I did the only thing I knew to do - I headed back to my office to work. But, I found out that I couldn't work in this state of mind. Shock was dropping by to pay me a visit - a very handy mechanism of the body that allows you to handle things before you lose it. Once I made it to the office, I knew I had to cancel my clients for the remainder of the day. I was in need of some shoulders to cry on. I sat down at my desk to call my sister and a few close friends to share the news.

Before heading home, I received a call from the nurse practitioner – the one who had written the referral for the mammogram. She informed me that the radiologist urged me not to waste any time in scheduling an appointment with a cancer specialist. I did not allow her scare tactics to overwhelm me. Instead I informed her that I would get back to them next week. I knew I needed some time to think things through thoroughly because my mind was a train wreck of thoughts and emotions.

It really just blows me away how the medical community immediately, upon diagnosis, tries to instill fear in you. In fact, everyone around me was reacting out of fear. Not one person thought to ask me what *I* wanted to do. I cannot express to you enough, do not get caught up in the fear! That is why I like to ask, "Is it fear or the disease?" Keep this thought in your heart as you continue to read the chapters ahead.

The diagnosis was delivered to me on Good Friday - a very significant day to all Christians. It was on this particular day that our Lord and Savior, Jesus Christ, died to bring us hope and a new life. *"He was wounded for our transgressions, He was bruised for our guilt and iniquities; the chastisement [needful to obtain peace and well-being for us] was upon Him and by His stripes [that wounded Him] we are healed and made whole."* (Isaiah 53: 5)

I would eventually see this day as a new beginning in the health of not only my body but also for my mind, spirit and soul. I knew I could be healed but, for me to get there, it

13

would be my faith that would become a very valuable commodity. What I needed right then - more than anything, was support and encouragement. I decide to call my dear friend Pam and ask her to stop by later on, knowing that she always came bearing gifts of good food and red wine. Yes, I still wanted to eat! Nothing kills my appetite - not even being diagnosed with cancer! Don't tell me that food isn't comforting. You can't take the Italian out of this girl!

Upon arriving home that afternoon, I called my friend Jan, who lives in California and who is a really strong Christian believer. I knew I needed to surround myself with people who would love me and offer positive reinforcement. She advised me to get in touch with a man named Eli and his wife Judy so they could pray and be in agreement for my healing.

Eli is an anointed man of God who has an incredible gift of healing. The Bible says *"Again, truly I tell you that if two of you on earth agree about anything that they ask for, it will be done for them by my Father in heaven."* Matthew 18:19 (NIV) I wasted no time in contacting them and asking them for prayer concerning my health. I found it so amazing that I could pick up the phone and call someone I didn't even know and have them stand in agreement with me for my healing. I cannot begin to tell you how special and important this was to me. Even though I was still in a state of shock, I knew - right at that very moment, my healing began.

As the news continued to spread, most of my friends just couldn't believe this was actually happening to me. I was the one who always ate organic, took my supplements religiously and exercised consistently. But, what we think is healthy just may not necessarily be so.

Before I knew it, there was a knock at the door and it was Pam with food, wine, some liquid minerals - and a new boyfriend. My friend Pam, what an awesome woman she is. She's a little blond New Zealander who is as passionate about health as I am. If you need Pam, she is always there. Sometimes she arrives so quickly that you would think she had transported herself (beam me up Pam). This time though, I remember thinking, "Wow, not the best time for to me to meet your new boyfriend!" The real kicker was that his wife had died a few years prior from, of all things - breast cancer, or, as I prefer to say, *from the treatment of breast cancer*.

So, here I was with this strange man staring at me in fear and probably reliving some terrible memories in his mind of his wife's journey with cancer. And here I was in shock and as white as a ghost trying to make him feel comfortable and at ease. But wait, wasn't I the one who was just diagnosed with breast cancer? We women are so nurturing. Even in the midst of my own crisis, I was trying to comfort someone else. It's just what we do. Once we all gathered ourselves together – both emotionally and physically, we ate, drank and discussed some natural ways of healing - and how passionate we were about them.

After bidding Pam and her new boyfriend goodbye, I went over to see my good friend, Gayle, and we sat on her balcony with our dogs, relaxing and enjoying the rest of the evening. As we sat there, we began to discuss my health. With absolutely no fear in her eyes, Gayle very calmly said the best thing a friend could have ever said, "Venus, you're going to be alright." She has been my friend, my cheerleader and a shoulder to cry on throughout this entire journey. What would I have done without her or any of my dear friends?

Finally, the moment came that evening when I was alone with nothing but my thoughts and the diagnosis that lingered so loudly in my head. I remember going to bed that night, cuddling up with my dog and crying. Iggy never sleeps on the bed with me but, that night, he must have known that I really needed him by my side. It would indeed prove to be a sleepless night.

Getting up around 4 a.m., I gave up the battle of trying to get some rest. I immediately found myself on the computer searching for any possible natural cures for breast cancer. I had no idea how this was going to change my life viewpoint of how I defined 'healthy'. I found more information on the benefits of eating raw, living foods than any other options. There have been times in my past that I have thoroughly enjoyed eating at raw food restaurants but I actually never thought about becoming a raw food enthusiast. Was I going to be a hippie again, wear dreadlocks and give the peace sign all day? Did I have to give up makeup, not shave my arm pits - or legs too?

By eating raw foods I mean mostly raw fruits, vegetables, nuts and seeds. The premise is that heating food destroys its nutrients and natural enzymes which is bad because enzymes boost digestion and fight chronic disease. Even enlightened doctors know that recent reputable studies suggest that food choices may affect the risk for recurrence and survival, especially for breast, colon and prostrate cancers.

I have been a vegetarian a couple of times in my life, however, I didn't really benefit from it as much as I could have because I consumed too many refined carbohydrates and soy products - which aren't actually healthy.

The information I was finding on the raw vegan diet was very appealing to me. The food can be as gourmet as you want it to be and is very flavorful as well. A raw vegan diet consists of no animal products, dairy, refined sugars, or gluten and the food is never heated above 115 degrees Fahrenheit. This method of preparation allows our foods to keep all of their enzymes, micro nutrients and antioxidants alive instead of depleting it of the nutrients we really need.

The Bible is very specific in telling us the importance of taking good care of our bodies. *"Do you know not that your body is a temple of the Holy Spirit, who is in you, whom you have received from God? You are not your own, you were bought with a price. Therefore honor God with your body."* (1 Corinthians 6:19-20) I really did - and still do, want to bring honor to God by taking care of my body. I decided to do better than I had in the past.

I made the commitment to give up sugar and to follow the raw vegan diet for the first six months after the diagnosis. After that period of time, I followed the raw vegan way of eating about 80 percent of the time, allowing myself the other 20 percent to add cooked foods that I felt my body needed. I also allowed myself to enjoy the occasional treat. I only ate raw desserts, though, because refined sugars could not be a part of my diet. Recipes and ideas for this raw diet can be found on my website and in my cookbook.

I learned that cancer cells do not breathe oxygen. They are anaerobic cells - *and they love sugar*. In fact, a cancer cell has six to thirteen times more insulin receptors than a healthy cell has because it is not breathing oxygen - it is fermenting sugar. It lights up the cancer cells, gives it energy and can multiply it.

One of the first things I had to do was to get my kitchen in order so I could begin preparing raw, living foods properly.

I needed to add some additional appliances besides the food processor I already owned. I invested a few bucks in a Vita Mix blender - the lawnmower of blenders. It can break down anything and is great for preparing green smoothies. The other two items I added were a good juicer and a dehydrator that have both done wonders for my health. I feel and look so much better since I have changed my way of preparing and eating food. I can honestly say that I have found the food to be absolutely delicious, filling and - most of all, very satisfying.

So, as God gave me wisdom and insight, I was successfully on my way to detoxing and healing my body. *"For skillful and godly Wisdom shall enter into your heart and knowledge shall be pleasant to you."* Proverbs 2:10 (Amp) I knew that this was a journey - not an overnight adventure. I was asking God to reveal His wisdom and knowledge to point me in the right direction every single step of the way.

I set aside time to educate myself about supplements to alkalize my body in order to reduce inflammation and kill cancer stem cells. I also added daily shots (not as in needles) of wheat-grass to my diet - removing my weekly shots of tequila. Let me repeat myself, this did not happen overnight. It is a journey. You cannot do something for two to three days - or even a week, and expect to get the results you are looking for - and need. Stick with it and I promise you will see results.

Back to the weekend I was diagnosed... I spent that Saturday in a complete daze. The next day - Easter Sunday, I was invited over to my friends Janelle and Kyle's home for our annual adult Easter party. Now, keep in mind that stress affects everyone very differently. After having a few cocktails (I had not arrived at the no alcohol state yet), I was feeling no pain. I know I was trying to cover up the excessive emotional pain I was carrying on the inside.

I found myself in the front yard hanging out when I decided, or should I say, I was determined to see the neighbor's - Tim and Damon's - two basset hounds. I asked Tim, "Can I see your dogs?" He said no because Damon had hurt his back and was resting. I don't have a clue as to what possessed me to do what I did at that moment but, right there in the front yard, I took my shirt off. "Does this change your mind?" I asked. He then reminded me that he was gay.

Stress does crazy things to people! Every Easter, my friends love to bring this up. They joke and say, "Yeah Venus, it's all about the Ta Ta's." I don't think I will ever live this one down.

My old habits were beginning to re-surface again. I was resorting to what I knew - drinking to de-stress and partying to cover up the pain. However, I knew that I had to make some serious changes in the way I was living my life. I have always loved the Lord, but there have been times in my life that I didn't include Him with me on my journey. I was reverting back to what I used to do - allowing my human-ness (flesh) to prevail, and I knew it was time to get myself together - *to get serious about this diagnosis*.

I am including all of me in this book - no matter how offensive or over the top it may seem, to keep things real. I realize that this book may not meet the so-called "proper" guidelines for some Christians, however, bear with me because I have decided that I am going to tell the raw truth about my experience - no matter what. I knew I had to deal with a lot of stuff before I was ready to get down to business with being healed.

So, nine days later,

April 19, 2009 *I am headed to Shoreline Church where I have been attending for about six months. As the service starts and the worship music begins, this overwhelming feeling of desperation begins to set in. I know I need something miraculous from God. The time comes in the service where they invite people who have requests to come forward to pray with the prayer partners. I have never done this before and it is completely out of my comfort zone. I realize - especially in the face of something like cancer, the importance of stepping outside of my comfort zone.*

I ask Gayle - who is sitting next to me, to go down and pray with me. As we approach the prayer partner, Gayle shares with her that the radiation machine (called a mammogram) has found a lump in my breast. All I can do is stand there and cry.

Returning to our seats, I feel an incredible amount of peace hovering over me and a calmness that is so welcoming.

On that day - I didn't realize it at the time, but I had met someone who would end up being very important to me on the journey that lay ahead - and I would have never met her if I had just stayed in my seat. Again I'll say, "Step out of your comfort zone!"

April 20, 2009 I am off to my first appointment with a cancer specialist and I just know that today is the day I am going to receive a clean bill of health. The waiting room is filled with somber faces, but - not me, I am with my friend Andrea Wells and we are - odd as it may seem, laughing and making jokes. If you haven't heard, the body can't heal without joy. I know you've heard before that laughter is the best medicine. It's true. "A happy heart is a good medicine and a cheerful mind works healing but a broken spirit dries up the bones." Proverbs 17:22 (Amp)

I know that I have to laugh and find joy in order for my body to heal.

The next thing I remember about that day is when the nurse called my name and led me to the examination room. I'd like to point out that I carefully selected a female doctor thinking that she would be much more compassionate than a male physician. Turns out, sex plays no part in the role of being a compassionate "*cancer doctor*."

Mistake number one, I allowed "*Dr. Do-little for me*" to do a needle biopsy which would be a decision that I would come to regret down the road. If I had only known what I know now, I would have never permitted this procedure to happen.

You see, a tumor is a calcified mass that encapsulates cancer cells to protect the body. Inside of a tumor can be cancer cells, but the tumor's surface itself is not cancerous. By sticking a needle into a tumor, it can cause the cancerous cells to spread throughout the body into the blood stream and lymph system therefore upping the chances of metastasizing the cancer. This is commonly referred to as tumor spillage. Metastasis is usually what ends up making cancer so deadly.

Before leaving, the doctor said she would call me with the pathology results as soon as they came in. She told me she was certain that the mass was cancerous, recommending a mastectomy and chemotherapy. I looked at her and firmly told her, "NO, you will not!" She completely ignored my response telling me to make an appointment with her nurse for a PET scan - which cost $2,000. It also has such an extreme amount of radiation that they advise you not to be around small children or pregnant women for a certain amount of time after having this procedure. Could I even go home and be around my dog?

The cancer specialist called me the next day to confirm that the test results were positive. Oh, and let me add that she left this detailed information on my voice mail. Isn't that illegal? She reminded me again to make an appointment for the PET scan. Why do doctors think you don't have any say over your own body and why did she keep pushing this in my face? Money? Power? Control? These were honestly the only answers I could come up with.

The next day I found myself Googling slang words for breasts. To my surprise I ended up writing down over 138 variations. For example: airbags, bazookas, boobs, chesticles, cupcakes, dairy pillows, devils' dumplings, fun bags, hooters, hood ornaments, jugs, knockers, rib bumpers, tits - and this is just to name a few of my favorites. We all love them; beautiful mounds of flesh, fat and glands. So, why would I want to lose them? They are a part of me and, yes, a part of being a woman - *whether they are AA or EE*. They are part of my God given body and I'm going to keep my Bodacious Ta Ta's.

I called and informed the not-so-compassionate doctor that she was fired. I refuse to be a dollar sign! Breast cancer is BIG money. Let me say it again, breast cancer is BIG money! Each breast cancer patient makes the medical field as much as $800,000 to $1 million dollars over the course of the disease. In reality, where is the incentive to find a cure for cancer? If getting well naturally makes doctors or hospitals very little money - and doesn't keep you sick and dependent upon them, then why would they even want to find a cure?

Three days later...

April 23, 2009 *I am an Esthetician with my own private skincare business. It is a typical workday for me, except for my roller coaster-like emotions. One minute I am slowly climbing to the top and the next I am plummeting to the bottom at break neck speed! It has been some kind of ride these past few weeks!*

This particular day, as I began preparing for my appointments, I remember being full of overwhelming anger and rage that this is happening to me. I am so mad that I take my arms and, with one big swipe, throw everything off my desk. Of course, immediately following, I proceeded to climb under my desk, curl up in a ball, and weep.

A few minutes later my client arrives for her appointment to find me still underneath my desk. Thank God she is someone who knows me. She keeps saying, "Venus, you don't have to work on me today." I insist that I have to.

The truth is that I can't afford not to work. My business was relatively new and who else would support me? What complete insanity, having to work while I was at the beginning of my healing journey. But, looking back, if I had retreated to a corner of my home and let everything go, I would have lost all my clients - and my business. This paints a vivid picture for me of the realities that individuals go through every day and I can honestly see how some of them wind up homeless in situations like these. If I hadn't pushed through and kept working and if it hadn't been for my friends who supported me emotionally, it could have been me. I can see it now, Iggy and I on the corner with a sign saying, "Lost everything to Fear - not the Disease." At least Iggy is cute. He would have enticed the people passing by to contribute to our cause.

The first thirty days after being diagnosed are the most crucial to receive the support of family and friends. Instead of my family coming right away, they decided to wait until I had surgery - assuming that I was going the conventional route. Family and friends... wake up! The emotional toll this has on a person is overwhelming and no one - absolutely no one, should have to face it alone. My mother, whom I love dearly, didn't even come to see me in the beginning when I needed her the most.

My mind was intoxicated and spinning with an array of emotions such as shock, fear, sadness, and denial. You are not at a place to make any major decisions regarding your health for the first thirty days after being diagnosed. I highly recommend that you find a nice relaxing place and go away to allow yourself to de-stress and detox before you make any final decisions. Surround yourself with people who love and support you. It is important that you separate yourself from fear - and the fear your loved ones have as well. Fear is frenzy, everybody feeds off of it and, when that happens, you can't think straight.

I continued to find the results of the diagnosis and the behavior of the medical field a hard pill for me to swallow. Many times I was on my knees crying hysterically. And yes, there were a lot of tears along the way. When you find someone trying to take something away from you, you wind up blaming. I blamed my breasts. One time I was in the shower and I recall this feeling of hate toward them, not wanting to touch or wash them. I blamed them for my pain. But logically, they had done nothing to cause this disease. In fact they were my friends. The cancer was not caused by my breasts. It was just a warning sign that there was a much bigger problem in my body. So, in a way, had the cancerous lumps not appeared, I would not have known that my body was fighting to save itself – and that I needed to help!

At this point of my journey, I had not yet learned to rest

and trust in God as I should. When feelings of isolation and fear would crowd my mind inside the four walls of my home, I would wind up on the floor crying and asking God for wisdom. Then, one night, something so mind-boggling occurred. As I was on my face and knees in a fetal position with Iggy by my side, I cried out to God telling him, "If this is what I have to walk through, then help me to make the very best of it."

A sudden calm came over me that hushed the fear and noise inside of my heart. At that moment, I heard God speak to me as if He were standing right beside me, "Child, you are going to write a book and take the fear out of others' hearts." I said, "Really God? Did I hear you correctly?" That was the furthest thing from my mind at that moment. Yet, instantly, I knew what the title of the book would be. Will anyone really believe what just happened to me?

I agreed to the challenge and asked God to put the right people in my path and provide me with the information I would need for the journey ahead. I was finally beginning to understand what others meant when they said God spoke to them. This was a pivotal turning point in which I decided - right then and there, to become a human guinea pig in order to find out what good - and bad, treatments were available for breast cancer. It would be a mission to discover the truth.

I contacted a modern cancer treatment facility in Texas that is supposed to be the "best of the best" and made an appointment for a second opinion. I was going to see what the all the fuss with this place was about. I also didn't want anyone to say that I was lying about the diagnosis I was given at my first appointment. Notice that I do not say *my* diagnosis or *my* breast cancer. I do not claim the diagnosis as *mine*, and I refuse to own it.

I knew I had a lot of research to do before my appointment. I didn't want to walk in blind but, rather instead, as educated as possible. You see, sometimes what you are being told is not always the truth. Even though I knew my body was telling me that I had cancerous lumps in my breast and the doctors were telling me that I had a diagnosis of breast cancer, I already knew I was healed.

May 10th, 2009 I am fully aware when I get to the cancer treatment center it will be a real test of my faith. It's Sunday morning and time for church. As service begins, I feel desperate even though I know the route that I am going to take. As they call the prayer partners forward, something comes over me. I am barreling down the aisle nearly pushing people out of my way. I am determined to get to the same prayer partner who had prayed for me last week.

Success.

She speaks to me and calls me by name. I am amazed that she remembers who I am. I tell her that the test results have been confirmed and the diagnosis is breast cancer. She looks at me and asks, "Venus, what are you afraid of?"

I am afraid of the doctors.

As we prayed that day, the peace that only comes from God was very present and real to me. *"And the peace of God, which transcends all understanding, will guard your hearts and your minds in Christ Jesus."*- Philippians 4:7 (NIV)   *"Thou wilt keep them in perfect peace whose mind is stayed on thee." -Isaiah 26:3*

For me it was an in and out thing, fear... no fear, fear... no fear. But when I wasn't fighting fear, I was almost elated. Whenever I prayed (or was prayed over), I always felt an incredible measure of peace and a sense of bravery that helped me in moving forward. If you haven't heard before, prayer really does work.

After the service I connected with Lisa, the prayer partner, to tell her what I had decided to do - I was going for a second opinion. She told me that when she prays for people, she doesn't usually blurt out such an insensitive question... "Venus, what are you so afraid of?" I told her that no one had asked me what I was afraid of before. Most people would assume that I was afraid of the disease but, in actuality, I was afraid of the doctors. God knew exactly what I needed that day and I am so thankful that He connected my paths with Lisa's. There was an instant bond between us. It was as though we had known each other a long time. I didn't want to take advantage of her, but I knew I needed her prayers and support.

She provided me with some resources that she felt might be helpful. One of the books she gave me was *Healed of Cancer* by Dodie Osteen. The book was a beautiful story about how God healed Dodie after being sent home with liver cancer and only two weeks to live. She chose not to accept the diagnosis and prayed for two solid years for a clean bill of health. It has been over thirty years and Dodie is still declaring the faithfulness of God!

I repeat this scripture every day, *Cancer Is "a curse of the law..."* - Deuteronomy 28:61 and, according to Galatians 3:13 *"Christ redeemed us from the curse of the law; therefore I am redeemed from cancer."* The word redeemed means *to pay off, to fulfill, to set free of ransom.* In other words, Jesus paid the debt on the cross for all diseases saving us from the curse of the law. I continue to repeat this every single day, all day long, knowing that this affliction will never come upon me again.

My faith was blind. Though my eyes could not yet see the results of my healing, I chose to put all my trust in God's faithfulness and allow Him to be my great Physician. *"We walk by faith, not by sight." – 2nd Corinthians 5:7* I knew that by doing this, I was going to be OK. That doesn't mean I didn't experience some very dark moments, I just didn't stay there. I would pull myself back up to stand firm in faith and be reminded of the hope that I have in Christ. I fully believed that my new life was on the horizon. Each step of this journey would indeed prove be a true test of my faith.

May 11th, 2009 Kris Carr is my new inspiration. I ran across a DVD she composed called Crazy Sexy Cancer. *She had been diagnosed with a rare, incurable cancer and was told by her doctors that there was nothing they could do. She went home, educated herself, and set out on a journey to discover everything she could about the natural approach to health and healing.*

How impressive! I thought, "I want to do what this 'healthy girl' is doing." She has not lost her hair or poisoned her body - and she's made it through challenges like detoxing her body and her spirit.

This is my confirmation. I've decided to take God's natural path for my healing.

I continued to read and educate myself with anything I could get my hands on. In the meantime, I corresponded with a lady named Lauren, who worked at T-Tapp. She said, "Venus I have met this amazing doctor who offers oxygen treatments to cancer patients and he looks just like Santa Claus." I immediately responded to the lead and contacted him. He listened very attentively as I shared my story with him and my plans to get a second opinion. He was a very caring man and he expressed his concerns to me about my going to the cancer treatment center. He was worried that I would just go along with whatever they told me to do. I told him not to worry and that he was definitely going to be my next stop after going to this facility in Texas. I reassured him that I was one strong, feisty Italian woman and I would be OK.

In retrospect, I now completely understand the concerns he had. He was afraid that when the doctors pressured me, I might give in and go the conventional route. But, I had to know what women went through when they were diagnosed. Why do women cut their breast off within forty-eight hours of being diagnosed? It didn't make sense to me.

I had no idea that this would be one of the hardest battles I would face because of all the things that would come against me. I think Satan and his little demons were jumping for joy when they heard I was going for a second opinion to this cancer center. *"We're going to get her, my little pretty and scare the pants off of her."* But, thank God for the strength, courage, and peace with which He constantly sustained me. ***"For I know the thoughts that I think toward you, says the Lord, thoughts of peace and not of evil, to give you a future and a hope." – Jeremiah 29:11***

Blind Faith

We look not at the things which are seen, but at the things which are unseen – 2nd Corinthians 4:18

May 12th *Why is it that some people get healed and others don't? Is their faith weak? Or does fear cause them to run into the arms of a doctor that is pressuring them with scare tactics? My faith is blind. I cannot see my healing, yet I believe that I am healed. I still see and feel the landmark where cancer has tried to set up camp on my breast. Yet I know, yet I trust, and yet I believe what I know to be true and that is God's faithfulness and the work that was completed at the cross. "We walk by faith not by sight." - II Corinthians 5:7*

Blind faith to me is a personal belief that does not rest on any logical or material proof. Though I cannot see the results yet, I believe I am healed. That's my story, and I am sticking to it.

I know that cancer is not from God. If Jesus died on the cross not only for our sins but for our sicknesses too, then how is it that we are sick? That doesn't make any sense to me. In Psalm 103:2 & 3 it says, *Bless the Lord, O my soul and all that is within me, bless His holy name! Bless the Lord, O my soul, and forget not all His benefits, He who forgives all your iniquities and He who heals all your diseases.* Have we forgotten the meaning of the cross? I want to remind you as you are reading this that every disease known to mankind was nailed to the cross and it is the cross of Jesus Christ that is the prescription to your sickness. If you don't believe Satan can cause disease then read the 13th chapter of Luke's Gospel account.

Even though I know many Christian women who really love the Lord dearly, I ask this question: Where is your faith? It appears to me that some put their faith in doctors instead of God. They say God will carry me through, but what does that really mean? That God is going to get them through the cruelty of cutting off body parts, the poisoning of chemo and the burning of radiation? This is where I get confused and I see this as a conflicting belief.

Why would you let someone harm you to get you better,

yet believe that God will heal you from the damage the doctors have done. Wouldn't it be easier to trust God from the beginning and not move ahead without Him? Perhaps if some women would have just waited thirty more days, they might have received their healing. I am not saying that conventional medicine has no benefits. What I am saying is that it also is filled with uncertainties and worth navigating with the help of the One who knows everything.

I have spoken to many women - both believers and non-believers, since being diagnosed. I have found that the majority of Christian women are not open to hearing what I have to say about conventional treatment vs. God's natural way of healing. It's the non-believers that are more open to the limitless possibilities of our God. Why is that ? Most cancer treatments today are usually part of a clinical 'trial' meaning that you are basically being used as a guinea pig anyway. I respect the years and years that doctors invest in their education and in their practices yet at the same time, I am not going to let them become my God.

And, remember, just because you see, hear or read something, it doesn't mean it's the truth. I could have looked at my deformed breast from the tumor and given up a long time ago. Instead, I consistently walked in blind faith for over two years. I have known and trusted God from the beginning that I was going to be OK. Yes, it would have been nice to see instant results, but it didn't happen that way for me. While God indeed does heal instantly at times, it is not always that way. Sometimes faith is a testing of time. Hebrews 11:1 says *"Now faith is confidence in what we hope for and assurance about what we do not see."*

It took over two years for Dodie Osteen to get her medical clean bill of health even though she believed she had already received her healing two years prior. She was sent home to die and given a couple of weeks to live. Thank God it has now been over thirty years since that diagnosis and she is still living life to its fullest. Remember, if it is true that God told me that I was going to write a book to take the fear out of others' hearts then it may be no accident that you are reading this right now. I have seen some people receive their miracle on the spot while watching others walk it out like me.

I believe one of the reasons that the tumor in my breast didn't dissolve to my eyesight immediately was because there was so much for me to learn. If you get results right away, you may not appreciate the other benefits that come to you during your journey of walking it out. I would have never learned the things I did nor met all the people I needed to meet or experience the beauty of forgiveness and healing in the way that I did. Now, God can use all the information He has poured into me to help others along the way. There was a bigger picture that I couldn't see when I was diagnosed. Part of faith is trusting God.

We live in a society that is driven by instant gratification. We get sick and we immediately run off to the doctor. Who knows how long the sickness has been growing, maybe for years. But, we want instant results - especially when it comes to cancer. We automatically hear the word "cancer" and we think it's a death sentence and the drama begins in our mind.

When you are first diagnosed, you can't run to the doctor every thirty days or even ninety days to check for change. No one sticks to a given protocol long enough. Over testing in a short period of time is one of the biggest mistakes I see others make. When you do this, it opens the door to fear, not to mention that some of the tests are very expensive and some even carry with them their own health risks.

I fully understand and comprehend the vastness that fear can play when you are first diagnosed. But, the strange thing is that I can't remember it anymore. Logically, I know that I was very scared in the beginning. But, God gave me a beautiful gift of peace that completely showered my heart and mind and took away every ounce of fear that was within me.

Looking back, it's really hard to believe that I can't actually remember the feelings of fear anymore. There were many times of great darkness in the beginning where fear tried to make a home in my mind, but I kept fighting it with the word of God. As my Pastor says, "Don't exchange what you do know for what you don't know." I knew that God said I was healed and I also knew the importance that nutrition would play to help me get better. So, I refused to exchange these two valuable things that I did know for anything I didn't know.

It took me a good solid year to arrive where I am today and it's so amazing to know that I do not have to ever experience that feeling of fear again. If you asked me to give you a comparison, I would say it reminded me of stories of childbirth - painful during labor, but you forget about the depth of the pain the second you are holding that beautiful child in your arms. That's how I feel about the fear. Press through the fear. Choose to trust God and I promise you will see the fruit of your labor.

When people tell me they have been diagnosed, the most important factor they need to know is - if you are walking in the light Jesus shines on your pathway, you will make sound decisions. Psalm 18:28 says *"For you cause my lamp to be lighted and to shine, the Lord my God enlightens my darkness."*

As Dr. Caroline Leaf, author of *Who Switched Off My Brain,* says, "98 percent of all disease comes from thoughts." Alex Lloyd, developer of *The Healing Codes,* agrees. Everyone has genes that lie dormant until a thought activates them. I'm not a big fan of genetic testing. But, the medical society is convincing women everywhere to be proactive to the possibility of genetics causing breast cancer. Women are making foolish decisions to butcher their bodies for no reason at all. They have allowed a doctor to plant a seed of concern into their minds producing a harvest of fear.

There are pro-active types of testing, such as Epigenetics, which will be able to give you a solution to a weakness in the body. This gives hope, not fear and desperation.

Removing your breast does not guarantee that you will not get cancer in other parts of your body. Your breasts didn't cause the disease in the first place. People who go the conventional way rarely change their poor lifestyles. They think the doctors do all of the work for them and they fail to discover the real root of the problem.

I met a woman at lunch the other day at my favorite raw food restaurant. She was wearing a Susan G. Komen shirt. I asked her "Did you have breast cancer?" She softly replied, "I did." I told her that I too had breast cancer and that I was in the process of writing a book about how I chose to take the natural route. She told me that they scared her so bad, she went the conventional route and is still having a difficult time getting over the removal of her breasts. She asked me if the feelings she had were normal and I said, "Of course they are."

When men are diagnosed with testicular cancer I am sure

they think about it a little while before they give up a testicle. Yet women Immediately give up their breasts without thinking about it first because somebody tells them that their breasts aren't important.

Our breasts are very Important parts of our sensuality. They keep our sweaters looking good, they are great 'weather girls', and you can nurse children with them. Breasts are a significant part of our bodies! The woman continued to share her story, telling me that she is now in the process of undergoing additional reconstructive surgery - which they keep messing up.

People do not understand that doctors know surgery, chemo, and radiation are not the cure for cancer. They are still saying one day there will be a cure. After fifty-five years, the conventional method of treatment only has a 5 percent survival rate. The only things they have improved upon is that the hospitals are nicer, the breast reconstructive surgery is better and they've added some drugs to prevent you from getting as sick during chemo treatments. Chemo is chemo Is chemo. Bottom line!

I realize that everybody has to make their own choice. But, the main point I want you to walk away with from my book is not to make any decisions based upon fear. Get educated. I have never felt healthier than I do now and, even though I am getting older, I feel so much younger. I sleep well, have a healthy appetite and love life!

Faith has been my most valuable asset. It has carried me through the difficult times. God is so faithful and He always comes through. I like to say that He's an 11:59 God and will show up on His time, not mine. I knew all along that I was going to be fine and I am so thankful that He showed me in the beginning through a dream that I would be healed before going for a second opinion to the Disneyland of cancer facilities.

Even though I knew this, what would I choose to believe during my adventure at the Disneyland cancer center? Would I put my trust in the doctor's report or in what God had shown me in a dream? Would I believe God's word that healing is one of His benefits and that the work was done at the cross? Or, would I believe a piece of paper that said I had cancer? Through all the difficult moments I faced, I chose to have blind faith. Although it wasn't always easy, and though I could not yet see my healing, I trusted God to fulfill His promise to me.

One day I was walking Iggy and saw a lady wearing a beautiful platinum ribbon that represented cancer. Now, let me be clear, you will never see me wearing anything that supports conventional cancer treatment and all the fear attached to it. I will stand with my sisters, every one of you - and give my support all along the way, but, no thank you, absolutely no badge for me.

I asked her, "Did you have cancer?" She said, "Yes, I had

colon cancer." When I tell people I went the natural route they look at me horrified. I can't quite understand the look in their eyes when I tell them what I chose to do. Either I am plain crazy or I am lying. This lady said to me that she never knew there were any other alternatives available to her. Doctors do not feel comfortable telling you the other routes you can take. Cancer is big business in the medical world. Hear me when I say, it is big business.

One day I do plan to design a necklace that will represent a nonprofit organization which I will start. It will have a charm on it that says, "Healed." Not survivor. Not victim. Not cut, poisoned or burned, but HEALED. When you go the natural route, you don't have to survive surgery, chemo, or radiation. The only thing I had to get through was some lifestyle changes and some much needed detox. Nor will you have to survive a near-death experience because you are not poisoning your body. The natural route builds the body up versus breaking it down. I am not a survivor - I am healed and restored by my Father in Heaven.

If we were really honest with ourselves, we would admit that we constantly eat poorly, consume way too much fast food, drink contaminated water, go to the doctor too much and are, as a nation, taking too many antibiotics and over-the-counter medications. The human body is a survival machine that can heal itself if given the right tools. I believe those "right tools" address the physical, emotional and spiritual parts of our being. I know people who have eaten perfectly every single day of their life, yet they were never healed. They failed to enjoy life, be grateful, and have fun. What caused them to get cancer and never heal? What was so deep down in their soul that broke their bodies down?

What people have to realize is that you have to get to the root of what caused the cancer or disease. There are physical and emotional traumas attached to disease that we stuff down and don't take the time to deal with. Cutting your breast off will not fix these issues. You must take responsibility for finding the root cause and deal with the cellular memory.

Women are the worst - walking around pretending that everything is OK. Then, there are those who are full of bitterness all the time. It's one extreme or the other.

I recently spoke to a lady who works in the home health care industry. She dreads - more than anything, when she has to work with older women because 95 percent of them are mean, hateful, grumpy and ungrateful. They are old and upset because they didn't live their life to its fullest or life didn't turn out the way they expected it to. We all have these high and sometimes false expectations about life.

I thought by now I would be married, have kids, be living

in my dream home and even have grandchildren. I had all these dreams and plans for myself, but none of them have happened yet. Life is to be fully lived. That's why I love animals so much. They live only in the now. They don't think about tomorrow. Maybe, that's why they are so loving and happy all the time.

We tend to be disappointed - a lot of the time, about how our lives turn out. Was I happy when I was diagnosed with cancer? Absolutely not. Was that the plan I had for my life? No. Was it God's plan for my life? Of course not, but when I was diagnosed I had to make a choice, was I going to be happy or bitter? I came to a quick conclusion that we are all on borrowed time. You never know when your time is going to end. We think if we look healthy, eat well and exercise, we're going to live forever. But, tomorrow we could get hit by a car. We are all on borrowed time and we have the choice to determine how we will live each day. I am going to live mine to the fullest!

I never once said, "Why me?" I did talk to God about my diagnosis and said, "If this is what has happened to me, then let's make the best of it." Yes, I needed to know why I got the disease - but not "Why me?" The one thing I have learned from this is that life is short and I better enjoy every single minute of it. I plan on being here until a ripe old age.

Unhappiness and bitterness are wasted feelings - just like guilt, anger, and jealousy. Even though we are human and will experience all of these emotions in our lives, it benefits us to get over them fast. God wants us to dwell and think on the beautiful things that happen in life. *"Finally, brothers, whatever is true, whatever is noble, whatever is right, whatever is pure, whatever is lovely, whatever is admirable—if anything is excellent or praiseworthy—think about such things." - Philippians 4:8*

I believe that breast cancer is also an issue of the heart. Most women I have interviewed during this time have told me they believe they got breast cancer because of the excessive stress in their lives - or from a bad relationship. I also found that some women were diagnosed in the midst of a divorce when their hearts were broken. As I continued to dig deeper, there were women who suffered from being abused physically, mentally or emotionally in their past, including myself.

In *The Healing Code* - one of my favorite books, it talks about breast cancer being an issue of trust and patience. If the person whom you love and trust the most violates you, a breaking of the trust occurs from that violation. This leaves the heart broken in many pieces and void of understanding. Friends, if you have a child that has been abused, you must address the issue immediately. No one took care of me when I was abused and I believe that broken heartiness never healed, leaving me to stuff it deep

46

down inside.

Satan likes our secrets to remain hidden because if we stuff it down, the end result produces unhealthy emotions, reactions and sickness. You've heard the old saying, "You're full of crap." Well, it's true and that's not just physically, but emotionally and spiritually too. If you knot up, everything inside you knots up.

If you don't deal with what really caused the disease, I believe that it can reoccur - regardless of the route you take to heal. You can juice all you want, take supplements, detox and even allow a doctor to cut, burn and poison you. None of these things deal with the root of the disease. Deal with the issues of the heart, the mind and the soul as well as taking great care of yourself physically.

My life has changed so much since the day I was diagnosed. I am grateful for the blessing it has turned out to be. It has made me look at things so differently. I have met so many wonderful people along the way, from doctors to researchers and individuals from all walks of life and all of them have played such an integral part in my journey. I can see my life's purpose so clearly now.

Being diagnosed allowed me to mend my ways and forgive my parents. It was learning and walking through the process of forgiveness that has allowed me to heal. If bad things have happened to you in your life, I want you to know that God can take those things and turn them into something beautiful. *"I will comfort all who mourn, and provide for those who grieve in Zion – I will bestow on them a crown of beauty instead of ashes, the oil of joy instead of mourning and a garment of praise instead of a spirit of despair." - Isaiah 61: 2-4*

I consistently speak life over myself and say I am healed. After two years, people still ask me, "How is your health Venus?" My reply is, "I am healed and my health is perfect. How about yours?" You have to claim and know that you are healed. This disease will never afflict me again - not in one year or even five years down the road. Conventional patients have that five-year window hanging over their heads which, to me, is five years of fear. The doctor knows that there is a significant chance of recurrence within the first five years.

Blind faith is like sowing a seed. The farmer cannot see the harvest with his eyes that lies in that tiny seed, yet he knows that if he waits patiently, the day will come when he will receive a beautiful harvest. I challenge you to do the same thing with your faith. Sow a tiny seed of trust in God and watch to see the results that will bloom right before your eyes.

Blind faith taught me to say my disease was over and that I was healed when I was diagnosed, I just didn't realize it. The debt was paid at the cross. *Christ suffered for us and left us an example so we can follow in His footsteps. "He who committed no sin, nor was deceit found in His mouth, He who, when He was reviled, did not revile in return, He who, when He suffered, He did not threaten but committed Himself fully to God who judges righteously. He bore our sins in His own body on the tree so that we, having died to sins, might live for righteousness and it is by His stripes we are healed* - I Peter 2:23-24

The magic pill for your disease is to walk in blind faith.

- Venus DeMarco

The Disneyland of Cancer Treatment Centers

May 18th, 2009 It's a Monday morning, my car is packed, and I am off to get a second opinion. I will be staying with a friend's mom, Virginia, who is a wonderful Christian woman living in Houston. As I get closer to her home, my car begins to act funny. How can this be? My car is less than a year old. I get one block from Virginia's home when my steering wheel column locks up and I realize that all of the power steering fluid has leaked out. As the tears begin to stream down my face and my body tenses with stress, I realize that the test of faith has begun.

Obviously, I was a bit rattled by the time I arrived at Virginia's home. But, as soon as I walked through her doors, I remember feeling a peace that lingered in the air. It quickly soothed my weary heart. After settling in, I make a quick call to Lisa, my prayer partner at Shoreline; to share a dream I had had the night before.

In my dream, a lightning bolt struck my breast. I was awakened by the brightness of the light in my room. It didn't scare me nor did I think much about what had happened, I just peacefully drifted back to sleep. Lisa said she would look up the meaning in a dream book she had and get back to me. But, we both knew without even checking that I had a visitation from God that night and He was showing me that I was healed.

Lisa phoned me later to confirm that lightning means sudden miracle. How amazing that God would give me confirmation in a dream, prior to everything I was about to go through, and tell me that I was healed. Even though the test that I was about to have would not say I was healed. Blind faith is what has sustained me. Sometimes the miracle is done, but you don't know it because you can't see it. What you see isn't the truth. From that night on, I vowed to be steadfast in my faith, trusting God that I was healed even though I couldn't see the results.

When morning came and it was time to get ready for my appointment, Virginia was preparing to leave for work. I said, "I can't go alone, and besides, I can't drive my car. Please go with me." Virginia was so gracious. She made a quick call into work and rearranged her day in order to take me to my appointment.

As we entered through the doors of the facility in Texas (that I call the Disneyland of cancer), we were greeted by the reeking smell of sickness. Though the facility was elaborately decorated, I found it to be a very demonic, infested place. The first series of appointments would take me to a floor where I would have my blood work and x-rays done. On display for our viewing pleasure was a lovely baby grand piano in the waiting room area. Soothing worship music would have helped to change the mood and atmosphere of this very dark place.

I really had no idea what was in store for me in the next few days. I literally gained ten pounds overnight due to the overwhelming stress I was feeling about my visit to the "theme park."

While there, I found myself being thoroughly interrogated by a nurse based upon the questionnaire I had completed before going into the examination room. She wanted to know why I was taking a supplement called Turmeric. I told her I wanted to protect myself from all the radiation that they were going to expose me to during my visit. She smugly replied, "Nutrition doesn't work." I looked at her and told her maybe she should try it. Remember, I am a feisty, Italian girl who is not a push-over when it comes to opinions.

They sent me off to meet with the oncologist, who was a very kind man. I begin to share with him the changes I had made in my diet. He said he understood why I felt so healthy because my blood work looked so good and then he said, "You're just not healthy in your breast." I said to him, "Then I am not healthy somewhere else in my body because my breasts didn't cause this. My poor breasts are developing an inferiority complex from all these accusations."

He laughed and then asked me a series of questions about my family history. He wanted to know if anyone else in my family had ever had breast cancer. Yes, my grandmother on my mom's side - and two aunts. I knew he was going to say that my breast cancer was genetic. He didn't but I knew he felt it was a contributing factor, however, I completely disagree. I believe that their breast cancer came from an unhealthy lifestyle.

Heavy drinking, eating a southern fried diet accompanied by a large dose of emotional stress is no prescription for healthy. At one point, my Grandmother remarried and chose to give up her kids. I am certain that this decision was one of regret, leaving my Grandmother filled with intense guilt and sadness. Besides, tell me why breast cancer is an epidemic now. What about 100 years ago? While we have come a long ways in understanding the role genes play in our bodies, you can't blame everything that is happening on them. In my opinion, my genes had very little - to nothing at all, to do with me receiving a diagnosis of breast cancer.

From the blood test results, the oncologist decided to cancel the CAT scan. Thank God! Do you know how much radiation is in a CAT scan? I would prefer to not do a CAT scan because of the radiation. Instead, I would prefer - and would consider, having a MRI. All these abbreviations. Just knowing what they mean takes some of the mystery – and fear, out of these procedures. CAT is short for Computerized Axial Tomography and MRI is short for Magnetic Resonance Imaging.

Surveys have suggested that many CAT Scans are unnecessarily requested by medical professionals. These scans come with an additional risk of cancer. It has been estimated that the radiation exposure from a full body scan is the same as standing 2.4 km (1.5 miles) away from the World War II atomic bomb blasts in Japan. (Wikipedia) Now that should be enough to change any one's mind and to think that doctors are regularly using radiation as a primary method of combating cancer cells.

Typical scan doses: Note: A rem is a large dose of radiation, so the millirem (mrem), which is one thousandth of a rem, is often used for calculating dosages of radiation received from medical x-rays. An acute whole-body dose of less than 50 rem is typically sub-clinical and will produce nothing other than blood changes. Amounts from 50 to 200 rem may cause illness but will rarely be fatal. Doses of 200 to 1,000 rem will probably cause serious illness with poor outlook at the upper end of the range. Doses of more than 1,000 rems are almost invariably fatal. In other words, a mammogram is equivalent to 1000 chest x-rays.

With this said, I was willing to let them do just about anything to me that day in order to confirm that the first doctor's diagnosis was accurate. I remember the strange look the doctor gave me when the nurse left the room and I said, "Don't look at me like I'm crazy." He replied, "I don't think you are crazy at all."

My day at the amusement park for cancer finally came to a close and boy was I ready to call it a day. Virginia and I drove back to her home to relax for the remainder of the evening.

May 19th, 2009 Morning came quickly and I am headed back to the "Cancerland" to have the mammogram done. Mark my words, I WILL NEVER HAVE ANOTHER MAMMOGRAM AGAIN!!! They are extremely dangerous, with concentrated amounts of radiation being shot into your breasts as they are compressed and flattened like pancakes between two metal plates. This procedure can damage the lymph system and aggravate the tumor, releasing cancerous cells throughout the entire body. There are alternatives to mammograms and I will discuss this later.

As soon as I walk into the room, I am greeted by the technician who says, "I was just praying for you before you arrived." I have never been squeezed, pressed, or turned in so many directions. I ask the technician if she has ever heard of miracles happening here. She replies, "Once there was a rumor that someone who supposedly had cancer returned for another test and the results showed no signs of the disease." She pauses. "You never have to do anything here that you don't want to do." Kind of odd I thought for her to say that...

After I was done with the mammogram, I was sent off to another place in the tall building to get an ultra sound. They had me wait in a strange little dressing room area with a curtain. As I sat there waiting... and waiting - *for over an hour*, I began to see employees leave for the day. At this point, the lady who had done my mammogram walks by and I remember complaining to her how long I had been sitting there. She never turns her body toward me - only her head, and says, "Remember, you don't have to do anything you don't want to do."

Finally, I get into the ultrasound room where, to my surprise, I have to wait another half hour. When the technician for the ultrasound does finally come in, she immediately engages in conversation with me about her son living in Austin. She tells me that he works at some juice bar and says he is "all into health and thinks 'that juicing stuff' works," to which I nicely say, "It really does."

I find it a bit surprising that doctors and those in the medical community don't even believe in the power of proper nutrition. If they do, it sure doesn't seem like it. As she starts to do the ultra sound, things begin to get very eerie. The radiologist comes into the exam room - which happens to be one of the darkest ultrasound rooms I have ever been in. It is completely dark - except for the light from the machine. I feel such a demonic presence.

The radiologist tells me some of the cells have spread from the first biopsy and then follows up by saying that she would like to do a very aggressive biopsy today to determine what type of cancer it is. I reply, "My doctor didn't prescribe that." She says it doesn't matter.

I know that if I let them do the aggressive biopsy it could metastasize the cancer right then and there. It doesn't matter what kind of cancer you have - or if you are stage 1 or stage 4. Cancer is cancer is cancer and metastasizing cancer is what kills people. For those of you who don't already know, metastasize is just a fancy word for 'travel'. In other words, once the cancer travels from its point of origin - and begins to set up camp in your liver or lungs or other vital organs. because of the aggressive poisoning, burning, and cutting done at this stage most patients are so tired and in so much pain, they can loose their will to live.

Then, clear as day, I hear a voice say, "Get up now, put your clothes on, and get out of here."

I wipe the gel off my breasts and leave immediately.

When I get out into the hallway, it is completely dark. No

one is left on floor. I look at my phone and see that Virginia has text-ed me. Glancing down at her text, it reads, "Something is really wrong. Get out of there now." I rush out as quickly as I can and jump into the car. I am pretty freaked at this point and ask Virginia if she will take me to Lakewood Church since it is also located in Houston and also because I had been reading Dodie Osteen's book, *Healed of Cancer*.

As we walk through the doors of the church we are greeted by the security guard who tells us we can walk around but asked us not to go into the sanctuary. He didn't want us in the sanctuary due to liability purposes and the dangers of not having all the lights on in the building. Like a little kid, guess where I went? Straight to the sanctuary.

As we are sitting there praying, a girl appears out of the blue. I find her behavior to be extremely odd. She keeps saying that Jesus is the lamb. And he has a very big head and shares with us that she had an out of body experience the last time she was here. I look at Virginia and say, "That's it. I have had enough. Let's get out of here."

Once we got outside, we both ask, "Where in the world did she come from?" Neither of us saw her enter the sanctuary.

Satan was having me followed.

Though the day was absolutely crazy, I was able to

experience what other women go through when they are desperately seeking answers for the diagnosis of breast cancer. You will not see me enter through the gates at the Disneyland of Cancer ever again! Instead, I am committed to researching every avenue I can in order to heal God's natural way.

May 20th, 2009 *My journey has come to an end here and I am ready to go home. As I sit at a local auto shop waiting for my car to be fixed, I realize that I have to take some time off of work and de-stress so that my heart rate will go back down. Pondering my next move, my sister calls. She tells me that the doctor from the treatment center is on the phone and is worried about me. Gee whiz, now they're tracking me down through my family.*

I call the doctor back. "Venus, what are you going to do?" he asks. I say, "I am heading to Myrtle Beach to see a doctor who specializes in oxygen treatments. I am going to heal by God's natural route."

He is freaked out but he knows he can't tell me what to do. So, instead, he asks that I call him and keep him posted on how things are going. I take down his cell phone number.

As I sit here today writing this book, I am looking at that number written on the back of his business card. I think, instead of a call, I will just send him a copy of my book. I still receive letters to this very day from the cancer treatment center asking if I am cancer free. What a crock! All they really wanted was every penny they could get from my insurance company - and they succeeded!

After all the new inventions in modern medicine, many studies that survey physicians show the success rate for the conventional method of treating breast cancer is still only 5 percent - even after all these years. Why would I choose 5 percent when I can choose the 100 percent success rate by going God's natural way?

I have worked in the skincare business for over thirty years and we were taught the importance of good nutrition. Knowing what I know about the human body, it's easy for me to choose God's way. I can't imagine burning my body with radiation, cutting my body parts off, or poisoning myself. I know that this will take a lot of work - and faith, but I am going to trust God to direct me on this journey to get healthy.

The first thing for me to remember during this journey is that God is still working behind the scenes and, regardless of what is seen or felt. I am healed!

When a brave person takes a stand, the spines of others are stiffened.

- Billy Graham

Redneck Riviera

May 21st, 2009 *Right now, my emotions are pretty well intact and I am feeling pretty upbeat, considering all I have been through. I am preparing for the next leg of my journey as I continue to gather more knowledge about God's natural way to heal.*

I know that I need to meet the doctor in Myrtle Beach, but my finances are extremely tight. I am concerned about meeting all my obligations but, thanks to an anonymous individual who so generously paid my rent, I can now go on this trip.

61

Note: Whoever you are - and if you are reading this book, thank you from the bottom of my heart for your gift. You have been a very important part of my journey and your gift was one of many miracles that I have received.

I love my sister very much but I needed her support right now more than she can ever imagine. I have been calling her over and over again - even trying to bribe her into meeting me in Myrtle Beach. It is even much closer to where she lives than Austin.

I was just diagnosed with breast cancer a little over a month ago and no one from my family has to come to see me yet. I am so frustrated with them that I even called my aunt to tell her how hurt I was and that I hated my family. (I don't really hate my family - I just hated their lack of support during this time.)

I felt like it shouldn't have taken so much convincing for my sister to come and support me and that she should have said, "You're going to be in Myrtle Beach? No problem. I will be there Venus."

She did agree to go and I was excited to see her – and the ocean!

Tuesday, May 26, 2009 *I am leaving on a jet plane headed to Myrtle Beach - better known as the Redneck Riviera, to meet the oxygenation doctor for the very first* *time and to hang out with my sister. I have no idea what to expect on this trip but I am praying to get great results from the oxygen bath treatments and to gather important information that will help me to heal.*

In case I have your stirred your curiosity, it's called the Redneck Riviera because it's as beautiful as the French Riviera yet it is one of the most affordable places to go in the good old South. Riviera is simply Italian for 'coastline'.

As for the doctor I will be meeting, well, he is the recipient of many awards and is known for his pioneering work in the realm of homeopathic treatment and work on the eradication of many devastating global ailments. He has over thirty years of experience and has dedicated much of his efforts to research. Partnering with a chemist/inventor, they have developed, tested and are now seeking FDA approval for the oxygenation system they call Liquid Prana.

One of my main reasons for wanting to meet him is to find out more about his oxygen treatment baths and how they work. Research shows that cancer cannot survive in an oxygenated environment because it's an anaerobic cell. These cells love sugar and thrive in a very acidic and non-oxygenated environment.

The bath treatments he and his chemist friend developed quickly floods the body with oxygen and I firmly believe this is what will keep the cancer from spreading throughout my body.

I was proactive in my healing from the very beginning and I know that cancer isn't always seen by scanning devices. Doctors frequently use the term 'micro-metastasis' now whereas it wasn't common to consider undetected cancer in the recent past. My goal is to not only heal the cancer they *can* see but also to get rid of it anywhere else it is trying to set up camp in my body.

Later that day *"Santa", as I like to endearingly call the doctor, greets me when I arrive today. (I sure hope he has brought me good health and well-being as an early Christmas present this year!) We come back to a beautiful home that is located on the beach and is owned by a man named Mark, who is being treated by Old St. Nick as well. Mark has generously allowed a few of Doc's patients to stay here during their treatments.*

Now that I'm settled in, I've been given a tall glass of Liquid Prana water to drink while I wait for my turn to take an oxygen treatment bath. Liquid Prana is unique in that, after enrichment with a proprietary technology, the water is super-oxygenated. When consumed, this water replenishes the body by enriching the cells with bio-available oxygen. In other words, in a form of oxygen that is available for the cells to repair themselves, thus making the body healthier and more energized. It also serves as an anti-pathogenic (meaning that it kills pathogens in the body).

This water is unbelievable! I can't get enough of it! I just keep drinking and drinking it even though I am not really all that thirsty. My body keeps saying that it wants more. It's very obvious to me that I needed the life source (oxygen) that is contained in this water.

My bath is ready. I jump right in to the large tub without checking the temperature of the water. Ouch! It is so hot that I immediately hop out. I call for someone to come help me and this man who has been diagnosed with prostate cancer - who is sitting on the couch in the living room, is so kind to come to my rescue. He quickly adjusts the temperature perfectly for me.

After that first bath treatment, I realize that I have not been this calm and relaxed in a long time. I can already see my stress levels going down. After what has been a long day, I climb into bed and drift off to sleep very quickly.

I slept like a baby that night - twelve solid hours. By the way, rest is vital to your healing. The oxygen contained within the water that I bathed in went right to work nourishing the cells that needed it and killing the cells that didn't like it. This is how the body repairs itself each day while we are sleeping so be sure to get enough zzz's.

Wednesday, May 27, 2009 *I'm starting to enjoy these baths. It's taken a while to get used to the regimen of what I am required to do. Sitting still for a solid hour isn't that easy in our fast-paced society. As I learn how to enjoy being still and to relax during these bath treatments, I read and meditate on the 40 healing scriptures from Dodie Osteen's book "Healed of Cancer." This helps me purify my mind and be reminded of God's faithfulness.*

We are made up of a body, soul (mind, will and emotions) and spirit. Healing needs to happen in all of these areas when you are diagnosed with an illness.

Tonight is dinner with the boys! Doc, as I learn Santa is called by others, is whipping up a yummy batch of curry chicken with his handsome sidekick Chef Mark. What a warm and friendly place this has turned out to be. Everyone here came to be healed, yet they are unselfishly willing to help one another in their time of need. What a beautiful picture of grace being extended and lived out.

The next morning, Thursday, would prove to be a very difficult morning for me. I cried a lot during my bath treatment that day. I know it was a much-needed cry. It is so easy to bottle up your feelings and just put on a happy face for everyone else. But, there's nothing like a good cry to help flush out and rid yourself of any negative emotions. Negative emotions get our body's vitals out of whack. There have been studies done that show that, after you stop crying, your body will move into a state of relaxation and your breathing and heart rate will return to normal as well.

__Thursday, May 28, 2009__ Today, I meet an amazing twelve-year-old girl who has such incredible insight and strength for her age. Her father, Vern, was diagnosed with stage 4 colon and liver cancer. He had surgery to remove parts of his colon but chose not to have chemo. There is less cancer now, but he still has three tumors left in his liver. She comes here with her mother so that her dad can get the oxygen bath treatments three times a day.

I ask her how they found Doc and she said that her dad was talking to a man named Ray at church about what was going on with his health and how he didn't know what to do. Ray told him about Mark's story of being healed from a potentially fatal Non Hodgkin's Lymphoma and contacted him to see if he would open up his home.

Within approximately two months of the treatments, her dad has witnessed healing taking place in her his body. When he first arrived, he had a lot of moles on his back that are now practically smooth and his face is clear. It seems the benefits of the increased oxygen go beyond just cancer.

I found out that before he started taking the bath treatments he didn't have much energy. Just recently he spent an entire day with his daughter watching her play tennis and then they went to the movies - and even hung out some more afterwards. He is able to enjoy doing things again.

Later *I'm starting to see the signs that my body is beginning to detoxify. My tonsils are swollen and my lymphatic system is moving stuff out. You know what they say, "Better out than in!"*

I call the Disneyland of Cancer treatment center to request that they fax my test results over to Doc so he can review them and share his recommendations for healing.

I never did hear back from the center. I think they may have been upset that they didn't receive any more insurance money from me and my Ta Ta's.

Later that night *Thank God that a friend of Doc's - Ms. Bonnie, brought us dinner tonight because these men eat like crap. While I was initially impressed by their food choices, I found out they only cook one good meal a day. Then, the rest of the day, they eat junk. Remember to do what your mom always taught you - eat your veggies. Nutrition is such a key factor in healing.*

Vern's wife (the twelve-year-old girl's mother) shared with me that they lost their second son in a car wreck. I can't

68

imagine how difficult it must be for a parent to lose a child or how hard It must be for them as they learn to cope and try to move on after such a tragedy. They both have a personal relationship with the Lord that I am sure has helped them deal with their grief and has also given them strength during Vern's health issues.

Vern's brother is actually a Pastor. No doubt they also look to him for spiritual reinforcement as well as encouragement. Like most of those who come into the home, they know that all things are possible with God. "Jesus looked at them and said, 'With man this is impossible, but with God all things are possible.' - Matthew 19:26 I don't know how people manage in everyday life or in a crisis without God. He gives me hope!

Friday, May 29, 2009 I can't believe it is Friday already! The week has just flown by. This morning I enjoy a cup of coffee with Doc as we overlook the ocean and I can honestly say it doesn't get much better than this. During my bath this morning, I read Dodie Osteen's book again. It always seems to help remind me of God's promises. Controlling your thought pattern during this time is crucial. You have to get rid of the fear that will try to inundate your mind. "For God did not give us a spirit of fear..." 2 Timothy 1:7

In other news, my sister is coming today and I can't wait

to see her. She has not seen me since I was diagnosed. Of course, of all the days I am supposed to enjoy time with her, today I am starting to not feel so well due to my body detoxing from the baths. Instead of staying at the house with 'the boys', we will be staying at a beautiful ocean view hotel while she is here. I must say, things are lot less expensive in the Redneck Riviera – an ocean view suite is just $140 a night.

After we check in, we head straight to the beach for some rest and relaxation. I love the smell of the ocean air, the sound of the waves rolling in and the sand between my toes. I also love a little drama from time to time. I have to warn you, I still hadn't yet given up the cocktails in my life by this time - and I probably had one too many that particular afternoon.

Later that day *My sister and I are visiting a little cozy beach bar to grab a couple of drinks. There is a group of good old Southern boys to our left who appear to be quite entertaining - and handsome. How can they resist two hot flirty Italian chicks like me and sis?*

I hear myself laughing a lot during our conversations with them. I just love to laugh and have fun. Besides, laughter is such good medicine. It helps to reduce your stress level and improves your mood. At this point, I can say I am in a very good mood!

One of the guys hands me his business card and, as I look it over, I notice his name is T.K. Brown. I'm quite curious what T.K. stands for. Rather than ask, I name him Titty Kent Brown - which I announce to the entire bar. His friends are cracking up - and so am I.

I must say I've always enjoyed a good laugh - even at myself. I told you this was a journey. I am sure that to this day, Titty Kent Brown is being harassed by his friends.

After our fun time with the boys at the beach, we head back to Mark's home so I can take my oxygen treatment bath. But, by the time I returned to the hotel, I am starting to run a fever with really bad chills. My sister is worried and upset but, after calling Doc, he says not to worry.

At some point during that evening in a conversation with my sister, I recall telling her I didn't want to die over and over again. She reassures me continually that I am not going to die. I am five years older than my younger sister and I can't tell you how grateful I was that she was by my side that night. There is a lot of mucus coming out of my body and the chills are so extreme that my sister has to keep getting up throughout the night to put more blankets on me.

The next day, Doc again reassures my sister and me, explaining that I am going through a detoxification process where the body is reacting to all of the pathogens that are being killed by the oxygenated water baths. The oxygen is also nourishing the billions of cells in my body as well as strengthening my immune system, giving it the ability to 'take the trash out'. He says all the symptoms I have are completely normal and assures us that this has nothing to do with my breasts. This is just my body getting rid of the junk so that I can heal. The treatments are causing my body to detox, which is so essential in my healing process. Everyone in the house is getting great results from the oxygen baths - including me.

Sunday, May 31, 2009 *I am taking my bath and I am completely burnt out at this point. I know that I am leaving tomorrow and my emotions are running on high. I am in the tub crying. What am I doing here? Am I crazy?*

I hear the Lord saying, "I told you I have already taken care of it. You are OK. Get on with it, have fun with your sister tonight. I've already take care of it."

What timing and affirmation to hear directly from God and that He would remind me again that He took care of my disease way back on the cross. My family may not have been here for me all along, but my Father in Heaven is here every step of the way. I feel so loved by Him! Words cannot describe the peace that I feel right now.

During the days at Myrtle Beach, I enjoyed time hanging out with my sister on the beach. In the evenings, we would stop by Mark's home for me to take my bath treatments, visit with the other guests and, on occasion, help clean up after those messy men.

At the end of our time there, my sister and I stopped by to say our goodbyes. This was extremely difficult for me to do since we had all grown so close in such a short period of time. I got to live with four men for a week - each of whom was so kind and loving. That trip was truly such a great experience for me!

Tuesday, June 1st, 2009 *I drove my sister to the airport this morning. I can't tell you how much I enjoyed my time with her. I am beginning to feel somewhat emotional as she leaves.*

After dropping her off, I head back to the hotel and find myself in the room - so aware of how lonely I feel. I wonder if I will have a hard time trying to board the plane with the flu-like symptoms I am experiencing from this detox process. Everyone is already freaked out because of the swine flu epidemic going on nationwide. There are even signs at the airport that read: "If you have flu-like symptoms, do not board the plane." But, I don't have the flu. I am just in a state of detox. Of course, I laugh to myself, if I tell people I am detoxing, they'll think I just got out of rehab.

I call my friend Elaine before trying to board the plane to ask her if my symptoms are normal. She reassures me that they are. I am so glad to have friends like her. You never know where you will meet friends in life. I met Elaine at a chocolate festival. She had a small company called Innocent Chocolate and I would give a piece to each of my clients after their facial. Sometimes I wondered if they didn't come more for her chocolate than for my facials!

My time and adventure at the Redneck Riviera has come to an end for now. I am so thankful to my sister who was there for me when I really needed her. As for all the men at the house, they were kind, caring, and respectful to me. They gave me a sense of security and forever impacted my life. My hat's off to the good ole Southern boys who made me laugh - even you Titty Kent Brown!

I wouldn't trade what I learned on this trip - including the detoxification process I had to go through to begin my healing process. I feel so blessed and I know I am moving in the right direction.

Even after arriving home, it took me a solid week to completely recover and start to feel better. The first round of detox was pretty intense.   But, thank God, every physical detox since then has been a lot easier with the exception of an emotional detox I went through - which is a whole other story I will get to shortly

"The road of life twists and turns and no two directions are ever the same. Yet our lessons come

from the journey, not the destination." Don Williams, Jr.

Mexico or Bust

June 7th, 2009 It has been a few months since I was diagnosed with breast cancer. I am eating right, taking the correct supplements plus downing my daily shots of wheatgrass and poop-in' like a big dog. That's what happens when you are drinking Green Smoothies and eating a veggie based diet. Lots of fiber keeps you extremely regular - if you know what I mean. I am consistently doing my T-Tapp workouts to improve my lymphatic system and walking a lot. I am feeling good about the things that I am doing to take care of myself now.

Thank God for my dog Iggy! He will not allow me to lock myself away from the rest of the world. He makes me take him for daily walks, which allows me to take in some good fresh air and a little sunshine. I want all the Vitamin D I can get.

There are a couple of things bugging me right now. Number one on the list is my hormones. They are completely out of whack! I am having a difficult time sleeping because the night sweats are completely out of control. I'm also having continuous hot flashes all day. This sucks! It's a red flag and big concern for me. The other thing I am struggling with is my emotions. I haven't gotten to the point of fully grasping that my body will heal itself, which leaves an avenue for fear to creep in at times. I am also exploring every possible piece of information I can get my hands on that may help me heal.

I remember, right around this time, that there was one day at work when I was giving one of my clients a facial and sharing some of my story and she said to me, "Oh my gosh! My best friend's father is a holistic doctor who specializes in natural cures for cancer." Isn't it amazing how God can put the right person in your life's path at the right time? The information she shared with me was extremely relevant for my journey and would prove to be a valuable piece that would help me to complete the puzzle of my healing story.

I immediately contacted the office of this doctor that she recommended and scheduled my first appointment with him. He has two office locations - one in San Angelo plus a wellness center in Acuna, Mexico that he shares with two other doctors. I will be meeting him in Del Rio, Texas (about a two hour drive from Austin) because the natural treatments they do for cancer are not allowed by the FDA in U.S. The patients for this center gather to meet in the town of Del Rio and then they travel across border together to go to the clinic.

I have never been to this part of Texas before so I contact a friend of mine, Kate, who is a native Texan. She is also not working at the time, giving her the freedom to 'be there' for me. She agrees to join me on this trip and is even willing to drive. That, in itself, is a Godsend since I, at this point, don't have the energy to drive for long periods of time - or to handle a lot of stress. Even the simplest things at this time tend to overwhelm me and my main goal is to minimize anything that will cause unhealthy stress.

July 4th Weekend 2009 *"On the road again, can't wait to get on the road again..." It's Mexico or bust ! The day to go to Mexico approaches so Kate and I leave for Del Rio the Sunday after the Fourth of July. During the drive, Kate tells me about this healer in Austin that she volunteers as a receptionist twice a week. She recommends that I check him out. My initial reaction to contacting him is surprisingly hesitant because of my beliefs. But, I take his information and consider touching base with him when we return to Austin. I am very open to discovering the truth and willing to consider meeting with anyone I feel may be helpful to me and my Ta Ta's.*

Del Rio is a very friendly border town with a lot of good

Mexican food. After checking into our hotel room, we decide to check out the town and also our options for dinner. We find two options, Mexican or fast food. Neither of these choices is well-suited for my special healing diet. However, instead of feeling guilty over food - which to me is worse than not eating something that's in your diet, I make the best choice I can with the options available.

July 6th, 2009 as the sun rises to kiss the morning with its beautiful rays, I wait with anticipation to see what the day holds for me and my bodacious Ta Ta's. I have no idea what to expect from my appointment or what the doctor will say. I don't even know what he looks like.

As I arrive at our meeting point, I see a tall and handsome man who has a voice like Rick Bayless. If you don't know who Rick Bayless is, he is an amazing TV chef with a show called 'Mexico, One Plate at a Time'. Wouldn't you know, that as soon as I hear his voice, I immediately start to crave Mexican food? Muy Bueno!

Even now, as I write this book, when I speak with this doctor on the phone, I get an intense craving for Mexican food.

The other patients (who had also gathered at the restaurant for appointments at the center) load into a van to travel together into Acuna, Mexico. Kate and I follow them in our car. I remember how overwhelmingly poverty-stricken the Mexican town was where the clinic is located. However, the clinic itself has an upbeat name and is actually a very beautiful Mexican-style building located right next to an orphanage.

Later that day *This clinic is a place of hope, health and healing. The staff has a unique approach to clinical medicine. Each patient is treated according to his or her individual concerns instead of receiving a "cookie cutter" treatment for a particular ailment. Conventional medicine has given up on patients like most of us but the word "incurable" does not daunt the staff of this clinic. They are not discouraged when some say, "But no one has ever gotten well from this disease." We are told that the patients here routinely recover from life-threatening or supposedly incurable diseases.*

Many people do not realize that diseases which are considered incurable in one country are sometimes successfully treated in another. For example, Chinese doctors use intravenous garlic extract to successfully treat viral meningitis. German, Russian, and Cuban doctors use intravenous ozone to kill viruses of all types. In England, homeopathic medicine is sometimes used in lieu of vaccinations and is also used to treat psychological disorders. In Asia, acupuncture is sometimes used as the sole anesthetic during surgery. In my opinion, having a global medical perspective is critical for those seeking the very best chance of recovery. This clinic here in Mexico adheres to that kind of a global perspective in the treatment of their patients.

I learn that they have no allegiance to any drug company, machine or latest gadget. They keep an open mind - but also a scientific filter, to find the best treatments possible for their patients. Statements like, "My headache started right after I got some dental work done," or "Ever since I started on that high blood pressure medicine, I just can't sleep," are key truths they use to determine the root of the problem. Unlike many doctors in the US, they take the time to listen and don't automatically discount even the smallest details of what we have to tell them.

I learn from their literature that here at the clinic their core values are listening to the patients and diligently searching for the latest research on all ailments. They then earnestly seeking to find and cure for the root of each of our problems.

Some of the therapies I see they include are:

Superior nutrition and supplementation (oral and IV)

Magnetic therapy

Oxygen therapy

Ozone therapy

Live cell therapy

An arsenal of various natural substances

And, when necessary, conventional therapies.

Continuing to read their literature, I see that they view diseases such as cancer, Parkinson, Lupus, heart failure and Lyme as whole body issues rather than as isolated problems.

The breakdown of a person's immune system, poor nutrition, poor elimination, lack of restful sleep, chronic stress, toxicity build up, pathogen burdens and a combination of all of the above result in more than your body can tolerate and systems start breaking down. Their treatments work at a cellular level to rehabilitate damaged cells and turn them back into healthy cells. Some treatments are designed to eliminate pathogens such as parasites, viruses, yeast, fungus and bacteria while others help cleanse and detoxify your body.

Later that evening *I find my doctor, Dr. Hines, to be a very brilliant and passionate man. I can tell he lives his life to help people. Also a pastor, he knows the Bible very well and has a very compassionate bedside manner. He is so dedicated to helping others with their health that he has driven from San Angelo to the clinic in Mexico every week for the past fifteen years.*

Since 1994, he has also served as the Director of Clinical Research for a clinic in Acuna, Mexico that specializes in the treatment of advanced degenerative diseases. In 2007, he established a clinic in San Angelo, Texas which uses nutrition, diet, and lifestyle management to normalize the function of the endocrine system (hormones). He just recently co-authored the book, *The Road to Health* with Laura Shroeder, which provides detailed - and effective, dietary strategies to restore normal gastrointestinal tract function, alleviate blood sugar deregulation and help with chronic fatigue.

My appointment lasted for three solid hours. During that time, he shared so much information with me that my brain was on overload. It was almost too much for me to take in and absorb. He also ran some blood tests and the results indicated that I had an overgrowth of fungus in my body and was very estrogen dominant He said that most cancers are actually fungus-related (which is why it's so important to be on natural anti-fungals like chaga mushrooms, wild oil of oregano and Pau D' Arco tea). These are just some of the natural anti-fungals. He also prescribed some heavy duty anti-fungal supplements for me.

The main objective for me in going to see him was to gather some more information on the IV Treatments and any other natural options they offered for treating cancer. I was not aware, on the front end, how much time would be required for these treatments. In spite of learning about the amazing success rates, and, after hearing the details of the treatment schedule - plus the costs, I knew I couldn't live in Del Rio at a hotel for the next six weeks.

I made the decision that this was not the best option for me at the time. The big drawback for me is that I am single, an owner of a new business and the only bread-winner of my household. I don't have the option to close down my business and drag my dog Iggy with me to Del Rio to live in a hotel for a month and a half. The important thing I gain from my visit with to the center in Mexico is that he discovered that I had a fungus in my body - another missing piece of the puzzle.

I appreciate his wealth of knowledge and he and his staff will forever be a part of my life and my healing journey. One suggestion he had for me was to find an infra-red sauna. I wasn't able to find one that I could use on a daily basis so I started doing hot Yoga. For those of you in the know, it's not Bikrim but it is effective and I can do it at a studio close to my home. Even though I only saw this particular doctor one time, I have stayed in contact with him and his lovely wife Sissy.

July 7th, 2009 *I learned a lot on this trip but it's now time to say, "Adios Mexico" and "Hola Austin!" Kate and I are on the road again... this time back to Austin. During one of our conversations, she tells me that her best friend's mom - whose name is Sunny - developed this product called Pomegranate Breast Oil. The formula has medicinal qualities and the capacity to fight abnormal cells in breast tissue. I love how – once again, God has put the right person - at the right time, on my path. This is another piece I will add to the puzzle when I return to Austin.*

"Trust in the Lord with all your heart and lean not on your own understanding; in all your ways submit to Him and He will make your paths straight." - *Proverbs 33:5 & 6*

Home Sweet Home

July 7th 2009 Dorothy, from the Wizard of Oz, said it so well, "There's no place like home. There's no place like home." Though I don't live in Kansas - or own a pair of red sparkly shoes, I want to go home! Not only do I sleep better in my own bed, but I miss my sidekick, Iggy.

During my visit with Dr. Hines in Mexico, not only did I learn about the specific treatments they have for cancer at their facility, but he imparted to me a wealth of knowledge. For instance, the correlation between fungus and cancer is interesting and once again, that's why it's so important to get sugar out of your diet. Fungus "Candida" love sugar.

But, I just couldn't imagine living in Del Rio for six weeks and crossing the border into Mexico every single day for holistic treatments. I truly felt that it was better for me to return home after my visit. A very important part of the journey is determining what works best for you and what you feel doesn't. I felt that going home was my best option.

July 8th, 2009 *Now that I am back in Austin, I find myself asking, "What am I going to do?" I know I have to keep moving forward. I decide to spend as much time as possible increasing my knowledge on the importance of consuming living foods. Keep in mind; it's only been few months since I was first diagnosed. Despite this, I am already implementing significant changes daily in my diet that I know are crucial to my physical well being.*

I am also investing a lot of money into food, juicing, supplements, books and CD'S. Plus, I am trying to determine the right foods to eat and the proper supplements to take. By the way, I learned that everybody has advice for you and it will be up to you to weigh out the value of others' input and sift the good from the bad.

One fun thing I did try was a raw-food cooking class. Proper preparation of food is important. Being careful to prepare it properly maintains all of the enzymes, micro-nutrients, and antioxidants. Most foods we consume are depleted of the nutrients that are so vital to our health.

When you hear the term 'raw food', immediately most of us will say, "No thank you." That's why I took this class. It's important that you enjoy the food you eat in order for it to become a permanent part of your lifestyle. I now thoroughly enjoy preparing raw-food meals for myself – and my friends! I am here to tell you, there are some of the most delicious - and filling, raw-food recipes for meals that will surprise you and your family.

As I continue to review things that might be beneficial to my health, I recall the information my friend Kate shared with me on the way home from our trip to Mexico (when she had mentioned that her best friend's mom had successfully developed a product called Pomegranate Breast Oil). I learn that it was developed to promote breast health and that the formula has medicinal qualities with a key ingredient called Ellagic acid and that it has the capacity to fight abnormal cells and contains mustard seed to help detox the breast tissue. It also contains a resin called amber which is beneficial.

I contact Sunny and share with her who I am and how I got her information. She is so passionate about the product that she agrees to stop by my office to share with me the details of the oil and how it works.

When she arrives, we get to know one another for a few minutes and then go into my facial room so she can show me how to properly use the Pomegranate Breast Oil. We both take off our tops and she demonstrates on herself a beautiful type of breast massage that she says will help promote lymphatic flow. Isn't this just every man's dream? Here we are, two women with our tops off, massaging our breasts. Don't get the wrong idea, though. We did it in a very specific way designed to stimulate lymphatic flow and detox the breasts. I didn't think anything of it - and it wasn't sexy to us at all. Again, let me stress, I was open to exploring every natural healing source that was available to me.

While she was demonstrating the massage technique, I started to cry. Mainly, I am crying because it is the first time I've touched my breast since the diagnosis. Breast cancer is such an emotional journey filled with intense fear - and all of the misconceptions. I blamed my breasts when they had nothing to do with this diagnosis. I realize that I had almost become obsessed with the tumor.

I bought some of the oil and also found out that Sunny is the founder of "The Gathering for Health" headquartered in Austin, Texas. We part ways and I can tell I have met another friend – and have found another piece of the puzzle for my healing journey.

The main message I want everyone to get, as they are reading this book, is the importance of being proactive with your health - especially when it comes to preventing cancer.

One of the many ways of doing that, I found, is to massage the breasts with this oil on a regular basis. The pomegranate oil rejuvenates the cells and the skin of the breast. I personally have incorporated this practice into my daily schedule and I believe that every woman should do the same.

July 9th, 2009 *When I said I would try anything, good or bad, well, I meant it. I scheduled an appointment to get a lymphatic massage. In case you are wondering exactly what that is, a lymphatic massage stimulates the lymph - a colorless fluid that travels through vessels in the lymphatic system and carries cells that help fight infection and disease. I explain to the female masseuse that I have been diagnosed with breast cancer and she insists on including a special treatment that will heal me. She holds this lovely crystal over me and lets it spin in circles. She says the crystal will draw the tumor out of my body. It's pretty amazing how many people think they can actually heal. I truly believe this woman's intentions were good, but I knew that a crystal is not going to heal me.*

Just a word of caution: Be careful who you see and what you do. Don't become so desperate that fear causes you to make foolish decisions. I am very fortunate not to have been swept away by some of the people – and practices, I found along my healing journey. I try to keep my family and friends in the loop of what I am doing. A solid foundation is a must! It's important to have a reliable sounding board and sometimes the only voice you can listen to is **His.** - **"If any of you lacks wisdom, ask God, who gives to all liberally and without reproach and it will be given to you. Be sure to ask in faith, with no doubting, for those who doubt are like waves of the sea, driven and tossed by the wind."** – **James 1:5-6**

Each week I continue to invest more money in my healing as I also spend more time researching and reading everything I can. I have been so inspired by listening to others share their stories. I ran across one lady who changed her diet to 100 percent raw food (no cooked foods whatsoever and no coffee) and was completely healed of breast cancer.

Speaking of coffee, if you have to drink it, I recommend Bulletproof or Longevity brands because they contain the fewest mycotoxins (fungus), they are organic and 7.2 on the PH scale. Also, dark roasted coffees are known to be less acidic (a good thing) than light roasted coffees which is beneficial in cutting down on extra acid that the body has to process.

As far as my healing journey goes, I know that I have made the right decision not to go the conventional route. I am finally at the point where I am sure that I have made the right decision. By faith, yes by faith, I know that my tumor will be completely dissolved and I will be healthy and whole.

"Home is the one place in all this world where hearts are sure of each other.

It is the place of confidence.

It is the place where we tear off that mask of guarded and suspicious coldness which the world forces us to wear in self-defense.

It's the place where we pour out the unreserved communications of full and confiding hearts.

It is the spot where expressions of tenderness gush out without any sensation of awkwardness and without any dread of ridicule."

- Frederick W. Robertson

A Year of Discovery

During the first year after my diagnosis, I learned so many things about cancer... about God... my faith... my emotions... my hormones... the importance of live food and so much more. If I can stress one other very critical thing, don't '*become*' your disease. Learn how to enjoy life along the journey - even when it's difficult. Remember, God is always working behind the scenes and, even though you cannot touch or see Him, realize He is there and learn not to rush ahead of Him.

August 2nd, 2009 What a time of discovery this has been! I spent this past year looking into good (and bad) options to treat breast cancer. I had mammograms, ultrasounds, blood tests, visited the Disneyland of Cancer treatment centers, detoxed multiple times and in multiple ways, experienced the benefits of oxygen bath treatments, crossed the border into Mexico. I also learned that cancer is a biological process affecting the entire body and is not something that you can just cut, poison, or burn to get rid of. Cancer has a switch. It can be turned on or off. I also discovered that cancer loves sugar and that everyone wants to be a healer. I am learning so much along the path of my healing journey.

The main thing is that, without God, I couldn't have done any of this. I would have never made it through the darkness. By His grace, He has upheld me. "Do not fear for I am with you. Do not be dismayed for I am your God. I will strengthen you and help you. I will uphold you with my own righteous right hand." - Isaiah 41:10

The more you educate yourself, the more knowledge you will have in making wise decisions. I am constantly learning about supplements, how to alkalize my body, how to reduce inflammation and how to kill cancer stem cells. Here is a summary list of the things that I implemented into my daily routine during the first year:

God and prayer:

Without God - and my faith in Him, I wouldn't have made it this far. Take time to find a local church

where others can support you along the journey.
"Because he loves me," says the Lord, "I will rescue him. I will protect him for he acknowledges my name. He will call on me and I will answer him. I will be with him in trouble. I will deliver him and honor him and show him my salvation."-Psalm 91:14-16

Juicing fruits and vegetables:

Juicing extracts all fiber from foods so, when drinking the juice, it is pulp free. When you juice, the resulting fluid is essentially pre-digested, meaning the nutrients go into the bloodstream immediately, bypassing the need for digestion. Due to it being in pure liquid form, juicing is an incredible way to feed our bodies, allowing them to absorb the nutrients far more easily - and in higher percentages. I like to start my day off with a green juice, but, remember, you can enjoy drinking tasty green juices all day long. When juicing, use more vegetables and less fruit. If you are sick, stick to just green juices in order to keep your sugar intake as low as possible.

Follow a vegan diet:

Follow a local, plant-based diet as much as possible. It's important to remove - or heavily reduce, the animal products in your diet. If you do choose to keep some animal products in your diet, keep it to a minimum and ensure they are completely organic, raised on sustainable farms and certified humane. Local farms are always the best. Or, just make it easy and try the vegetarian way of life and eat a plant-based diet.

Daily shots of wheat grass:

Not only will wheat grass boost your health, but it will detox the liver, purify the blood, and aid in keeping the colon clean. Like most plants, it contains chlorophyll, amino acids, minerals, vitamins, and enzymes. Even though it is made from wheat stalks, there are no seeds involved so it is gluten-free. Wheatgrass is a good source of potassium, a very good source of dietary fiber, vitamin A, vitamin C, vitamin E (alpha tocopherol), vitamin K, thiamin, riboflavin, niacin, vitamin B6, pantothenic acid, iron, zinc, copper, manganese and selenium. The vitamin and mineral is roughly equivalent to that of dark leafy vegetables so it is a healthy addition to your overall health, wellness and prevention plan.

Green smoothies:

Green smoothies are when you blend your fruits and vegetables together in a high-speed blender, such as the Vita Mix. All green leafy greens have cell walls mainly built of cellulose. These are very difficult for our bodies to break down to access the dense nutrition the greens supply. Since most people do not sit and chew their greens until they are juiced, blending the greens with the blender allows the machine to do most of the chewing and makes the nutrients more accessible to the body. These nutrients will provide your body with the food it needs to heal itself. I know what some of you might be saying, "Yuck, I am not drinking anything green!" Just try it. You will be pleasantly surprised at how good they can taste – and how good you will feel !

Natural supplementation:

Supplementation is the use of supplements to stimulate your immune system and build the body back up. These include supplements that prevent or reduce inflammation, supplements that serve as antioxidants, and supplements such as different herbs that are known to kill cancer stem cells or get rid of excessive (bad) estrogen in the body. Essentially a supplement is something you are taking to help (or boost) your body so it can be as healthy as possible. There isn't enough space here to do justice to how important they are so I really go into detail on my website. I even recommend my favorite brands and have a store on there where you can buy them!

Pomegranate breast oil:

I added the lymphatic massage and oil twice daily which promotes breast health. I really feel this is also a great way to stay in touch with your breast health as you will more easily notice changes such as lumps that develop if you make this a daily exercise.

Getting my hormones in balance:

Hormones impact your body at the cellular level and your overall health depends on maintaining healthy cells. Get those hormones in check. This is such a detailed subject that the medical field trains doctors who specialize in this area of the body. Find a good holistic or conventional doctor who will measure them and learn how to safely adjust their levels so they will be your friend, not your foe. Some of the most prestigious doctors and researchers in the world believe that breast cancer may primarily be a disease caused by hormonal imbalance.

Balanced my emotions:

When the negative thoughts begin to race through your mind, take control of them and replace them with positive things. Reading the scripture verses in Dodie Osteen's book, *Healed of Cancer,* helped me to start replacing the wrong thoughts with words of hope and healing.

Remove as much stress from your life as possible. Keep short accounts with people and forgive quickly. If there is anything or anyone who is causing you extreme anxiety, I suggest taking a break from that environment or individual until you are in a healthy state to address the situation better. Your health is a priority.

Rest:

Even God rested after the sixth day of creation. The body repairs itself while we sleep, which helps us to fight off sickness. It is crucial to get at least seven to nine hours of sleep a night. *"When thou liest down, thou shalt not be afraid: yea, thou shalt lie down, and thy sleep shall be sweet." - Proverb 3:24* *"Jesus said unto them, 'Come ye yourselves apart into a desert place and rest a while.' - Mark 6:31*

Exercise:

It's a great thing to keep your body active, to sweat and get your circulatory and lymphatic system moving. Our bodies were designed to be in motion and the term 'use it or lose it' is so true.

I know that I have shared a lot of information with you. You do not have to do everything at once. I suggest that you start with one or two things and gradually add more when you are ready. Let me repeat myself: This did not happen overnight. It is a journey. Consistency is the most important thing you can do for yourself when making positive changes. You cannot do something for two to three days or even a week and expect to get the full results you are looking for - and need. Stick with it and I promise you that you will see the rewards of your labor.

August 18, 2009 It hasn't been that long since I was first diagnosed and I know that I am moving in the right direction. Some friends visited me that I haven't see in a while and they were surprised to see that I looked better than when they last saw me - which was about five years ago. They kept saying, "This is not what I thought people look like when they have been diagnosed with breast cancer." Those around me are starting to have that 'aha!' moment and are beginning to realize that you don't have to brutally poison, burn or mutilate yourself to get better. Healing comes from God. He designed our bodies to heal themselves, just look at the way a cut miraculously goes away if you give it time and keep it clean. Nutrition is just a bonus for you to live a longer, healthier life. I don't know about you, but when I am ninety-nine, I want to be in my right mind and full of energy.

As I continue to tell others that I am doing this the natural way, some think it is great - and others don't. It's funny how, after several months of my intense efforts to pursue healing naturally, others are starting to no longer question why I am doing it this way. The truth speaks louder than lies.

I say 'intense' because it does take commitment and there have also been some moments where I have been engulfed with fear. But, when I wasn't fearful, I was almost euphoric. I knew without a doubt that I am walking this out with God by my side. I tell everyone what He has done for me. I want others to know that my God heals and that there are other options to treat cancer *besides the conventional methods.*

Take time to discover the truth about your situation. Don't just believe everything you hear - even if it comes from a doctor. It's your job to be diligent in doing the research.

Discovery is the process of learning something, it is the fact - or process, of finding out about something for the first time.

Everybody wants to be a Healer

October 3rd, 2009 I stand firm in knowing that I have the right to choose what is best for my body. I do not have to forfeit my rights into the hands of a physician. This is a lot for me to process - plus I am still dealing with a lot of fear. Though I am fully aware of what the truth is - and I believe that God heals, I also find myself grasping for straws and then I do something that is completely fear based. I decide to contact the healer my friend told me about during our trip to Mexico.

I've searched all over for his phone number, but I can't find it.

(later in the day) I was doing a little grocery shopping and, as soon as I got back into my car, surprisingly there *was the healer's number lying on the passenger seat. My initial reaction was that this is a sign from God! I tell myself that even if it's not a sign, maybe He just wants me to experience this for myself in order to share what works and what doesn't. I am willing to do that. I make an appointment.*

October 27th, 2009 I am setting out on my adventure to see what the fuss is all about. The healer's practice is located in a rented office space and those who come to see him are asked to make a donation for their healing appointments. I find him to be very humorous and extremely personable. Sitting on the table next to him is a picture of Jesus and I think to myself, "This is a good sign. Maybe he's actually a Christian."

As my session begins, he puts his hand over my breast - not touching it, and I can feel the heat from his hands. He then tells me that he heals through angels and that we need to meet three times a week for the next six weeks in order for me to be fully healed. Logically, I think to myself, if he is an anointed healer, he could just lay hands on me and - right then and there, I would be healed instantly.

That night I was really sick. When I told him what had happened, he said, "It's a good sign." and "That is your body detoxing." Honestly, to this day, I don't really know what was wrong with me that particular evening.

November 2nd, 2009   I am sitting in the waiting room for my next appointment with the healer. There are a variety of people from all walks of life that are hoping this man will be able to heal them. He always uses the phrase, "I will heal you," instead of acknowledging that it is a gift from God or that God is working through him. It's is all about what 'he' can do rather than what God can.

I've started watching Christian men and women who are anointed healers on TV - and online, which helped me to better understand healing from a biblical standpoint. I have not yet seen an anointed man or woman of God heal in person. I do believe that Jesus heals and that He can work through mankind to do so, but men or women cannot, in and of themselves, heal alone. God has commissioned each of us to be His disciples and to go into the world declaring His glory. "And he said unto them, 'Go ye into all the world and preach the gospel to every creature. He that believes and is baptized shall be saved, but he that believes not shall be damned. And one of the signs that shall follow them that believe is that they shall lay hands on the sick, and they shall recover." - Mark 16:15-18

Later that month I have been consistently going to this healer during the month of November and I am still not *healed. During one of my visits, he made the crazy statement, "If you get pregnant, the cancer will go away." I thought, "This is absolutely absurd, because people get cancer even when they are pregnant. What in the world is he thinking?"*

During this month of seeing him, he had moved into a new office space and I finally realized what was going on. His new decor included Buddha, the Indian god Lakshmi, pictures of yoga gurus, big crystals plus, of course, a picture of Jesus. I started to understand that I was in the office of a metaphysical healer, one who groups Jesus along with all of the other gods and healers. Surprisingly, even though I was more aware of his beliefs, I continued to see him.

During one visit, my curiosity began to stir and I started asking him questions about the angels he heals through and if he could describe them to me. He said sometimes he has to ask them to leave because they distract him and take his focus away. Things were just getting crazier and crazier. I was so amazed at how busy this man was - plus how many people were willing to donate money in order for him to build a healing center.

I always avoided the group sessions because I knew that some of the people would be too much for me. But, one day, the only appointment I could get was with a group session. You can't tell me that God doesn't have a great sense of humor because He was willing to let me go one step further before He stopped all this nonsense.

As I entered into the room, everyone was gathered in a horseshoe shape sitting with the healer sitting at the front. All of us were lined up as he began his healing ritual and it was at this point, we all started getting hot. The 'healer' could perform his ritual and talk at the same time so, as things continued, I find myself caught up in the moment as I began to hear him make fun of a local pastor. As he is "healing" us, he begins making fun of this Baptist pastor by saying that his nose and face were red as some of others around me began to chime in and make remarks saying he is probably an alcoholic. The healer also said that he was going to buy his church building.

It made me so angry the way he was talking about this man of God that I looked at him and said, "Maybe he has rosacea." Then the lady closest to me says, "Yeah, I'm a witch and I thought I was supposed to burn up when I walk into a church. Well I've never burned." Someone else made a comment about the Ft. Hood shootings and how the military was to blame for the gunman's actions. All of a sudden, all the witches started to come out and one deridingly asked, "Yeah, what does give us this day our daily bread mean?"

It was at this moment that I became as cold as ice. It was like I was covered in dry ice. I was freezing. I was completely separated from the group. I knew that God was saying "Venus, this is your last time and I have separated you from them."

It was obvious that the healer knew something had happened because he kept looking at me and I could sense he was very uncomfortable. I didn't even care. There was a boldness that had come over me and I was not backing down. I believe in the supernatural too - my God and the healer's demon were having it out. Guess who won!?!

As the healing session ended, I waited for the healer. I wanted to give him a piece of my mind. He tried hard to avoid me and told me he was in a hurry but I was not letting him get away from me. I asked him why he would tell this friend of mine in the group, who was very ill and who already has an illegitimate, handicapped child that if she got pregnant, she would get healed. I said to him, "Do you know what you could have done to her life if she took your advice?" I went on to tell him that he had to take responsibility for his actions. He laughed and said, "I tell women who are in their seventies to get pregnant." I continued to tell him that he was not very responsible. He couldn't wait to get away from me. Eventually, he scurried off to his office to be with all of his false gods.

As soon as I got home, I called my friend who told me about the healer, Kate, and told her what had happened. She said, "Only the healer has the power to end a session and separate you from the group." That was a creepy thing to say – and also a lie of the Devil. I assured her that God decided to end the session on His time schedule and that He is in charge of my life. I let her know that when God says it's over, it's over. I also made sure she knew that I was never going back to see him again.

I have to admit, I'm a bit embarrassed that I told people about this guy because this supposed "healer" and his "healing center" is not of God. The truth is that Jesus is only true HEALER. I already knew this truth in my heart but fear was driving me to do and try other things that I normally wouldn't do. I am thankful that God allowed me to go there so that I can see what others who are looking for healing do when they are desperate – or deceived. Satan is subtle and that's why it is so important to stay close to God. I am thankful that He woke me up to see how the other side works and the lies that people fall for. I'm also so thankful that He took me out of that whole crazy ordeal just in the nick of time and said, "You've seen enough."

Still searching for answers, I am walking with Iggy one day and I ask God for a sign to show me that I was on the right path. Psalm 23:2 dropped in my heart. As soon as I finish my walk, I immediately open my Bible to find the verse. "He makes me lie down in green pastures; he leads *me beside quiet waters."* I knew God was telling me - and reminding me, not to worry. He was telling me that He was restoring me and that He would fulfill His word. The verse He gave me is from the 23rd Psalm and written by the shepherd boy who became king – David. Here it is so you can enjoy it. I find it so comforting and can see why it is often called the 'Shepherd's Psalm.'

Psalm 23

"The Lord is my shepherd, I lack nothing. He makes me lie down in green pastures, he leads me beside quiet waters, He refreshes my soul. He guides me along the right paths for His name's sake. Yes, even though I walk through the darkest valley, I will fear no evil for You are with me; Your rod and Your staff, they comfort me. You prepare a table before me in the presence of my enemies. You anoint my head with oil; my cup overflows. Surely goodness and love and mercy will follow me all the days of my life, and I will dwell in the house of the Lord forever."

If you have been diagnosed with cancer - and fear is trying to consume you, I want you to know that God restores. He refreshes. And He heals. Don't allow fear to take flight in your heart and mind. Instead allow Him to lead you beside still waters and He will quiet your heart.

There is only one God and one Healer and I can testify to His faithfulness. He is real and He does, indeed, heal!

"I am the way, the truth, and the life. No one comes to the Father except through me." Jesus, in John14:6

"I haven't seen you in a while, yet I often imagine all your expressions.

I haven't spoken to you recently, but many times I hear your thoughts.

Good friends must not always be together in order to be friends for it is that feeling of oneness - even when they are distant, that proves their friendship is lasting."

July 1st, 2010

I love Austin!

I know I keep saying it over and over again but I really do love this place. When something like cancer strikes, you find out quickly who your real friends are. I feel so blessed to have such incredible friends - both locally and across the United States, who have been by my side each step of the way. There have been days when someone would just call to say hello or to offer a word of encouragement that would brighten my day. Others took time out of their busy schedules to drop by for a visit or to show their care and concern. To all my friends who stood in the gap for me, I love you and I want you to know how much your friendship means to me. "One who wants to have friends must show themselves to be friendly. There is a friend who sticks closer than even a brother or sister." - Proverbs 18:24

You see, I found cancer to be a very lonely disease, especially in the beginning when I was trying to figure things out. At least it was for me.

But, let me tell you about the Ta Ta Sisterhood. My friend Janelle - who looks like a tall, sexy Shirley Temple, is what I call a 'super-friend'. She is someone who is always there for you and has a very special way of gathering people together. That's why I have given her the name, Saint Janelle.

After a year of exploring all of the good (and bad) treatments available for breast cancer - and being a human guinea pig, my money was running out and debt was piling up. Saint Janelle - and a group of women called the *Femtastics*, decide to rally together and host a fundraising event just for me. The *Femtastics* is a group I joined to meet new people, develop new relationships and network.

I had such mixed emotions about allowing the Ta Ta Sisterhood to do this for me. I knew that I needed financial help - and that I also wanted to get the message out that there are other options for those who are diagnosed with breast cancer, yet I was worried - and a bit embarrassed about what other people would think. While I was passionate and excited about others learning that there are other options available to them, I was concerned if anyone would actually show up for the event.

I had always been the one to give to others so learning to receive from others was a hard lesson for me. God was teaching me that there are seasons in life when we need to enjoy receiving. If someone offers to give you something, don't steal their blessing away by not graciously accepting their gift with a heart of gratitude.

With great anticipation, the day of the Ta Ta Sisterhood fundraiser finally arrives! I am so excited I can hardly contain myself. My prayer is for me to have the grace to handle myself well and share the message God has put on my heart. This is going to be one of the best days of my life! It is time to put my 'receiver' on! I selected a really cute dress and smashing pair of sandals for the event. Just a quick side note – rayon and polyester blend (no matter how cute) are not a good idea in the summer heat of Texas. The material doesn't breathe and all you do is sweat. You don't just perspire, you sweat!

I was completely overwhelmed with emotions as I arrived at the event. The Ta Ta Sisterhood knows how to throw one heck of a party and this was the first fundraising event they had ever done. 'Three snaps up in a circle' for The Ta Ta Sisterhood ! They thought of everything from food to live music along with a silent and a live auction – they even had entertainment for the kids. My wonderful friends from out of town - Victor, Shelly and Ellen also made the trip to be there and celebrate with me. My sweet neighbor Cambi came with her mother and aunt (I love her family so much!) Her mom, Cindy, was 'there for me' a year ago when I was in a car accident (right before I was leaving for Mexico). She is so kind and comforting. She just hugged me and let me weep. Thank-you Cindy! Friends I hadn't seen in years came out to support me. I couldn't believe how many showed up - even many that didn't know me. Joel McColl, Lorrie Sanger and the Sarah Pierce Band kept the place jamming with some great music all throughout the evening. As I think back on this day, I still get overwhelmed with emotion. This event had It all - from food to friends and entertainment - not to mention what a huge financial blessing it was to me. I have never felt so loved and encouraged.

As I am chatting with everyone and taking pictures, I realize that many actually think I have gone the conventional route. I'm sure they wonder why I have hair and look so healthy.

By now, I'm chomping at the bit and I can't wait to speak to everyone all at one time. It will be a great opportunity to let them know that I chose the natural way and to share with them my amazing journey and how God has been with me every step of the way. This will also be the very first time for me to speak in front of a group about my healing journey and to share what is on my heart. Looking back, I feel that those next 15 minutes were the start of something great. It felt so good! This is right where I want to be - in front of people, telling my truth, sharing God's truth and giving them hope while letting them see that you can heal without cutting, poisoning, or burning your body. If just one person walks away with the truth then, to me, it is a success.

After the fundraiser concluded that night, I went home and stayed up for hours talking to my dear friend Victor. Everything was still so surreal. Never had anyone done something so significant for me as this. When I finally went to bed, all I could think about was the upcoming speech I was going to give at a retreat in a few weeks. You see, my good friend Teresa Tapp - who has a dynamic company promoting health and wellness, was putting on an event she calls her T-Tapp retreat in sunny Florida. She loves my story so much she invited me to speak to those who are attending. I decided to call my speech, "Is It Fear Or The Disease?"

Would I choke and not be able to speak in front of others? Would they cry - or laugh? Could I get my message across to them about the seriousness of taking care of their health? I sure hoped so. These questions went through my mind as I drifted off to sleep. One thing I knew, though - without a doubt, was that God had called me to share the truth with others. He was so good to me to have surrounded me with so many friends and to the Ta Ta Sisterhood and the Femtastics, I love you! I felt so loved.

Friends, there are nothing like them!

"Friends are like bras - close to your heart and there for support."

"A true friend knows the song in my heart and sings it to me when my memory fails." **- Donne Roberts**

Defeating Your Goliaths

June 21st, 2010. Today is the day that I begin this chapter about my battle with my own personal Goliath. I've gone back and forth about whether to share this very personal, private information in this book, but I honestly believe that, in order to be healed, we have to be healed emotionally as well as physically. So, with tears streaming down my face, I'm going to tell you about it.

Before I do though, I want to mention how, even in the midst of a beautiful event like my fundraiser, there are situations that will try to steal your joy. Little did I know, while at the event, that someone had walked away upset with me.

This happens to all of us. Someone is always trying to

steal our thunder or our joy. If we believe the Bible, it says that we have no flesh and blood enemies so, in reality, Satan uses situations and people to try and snatch away God's blessings. The day after the beautiful fundraiser that the Ta Ta Sisterhood and the Femtastics put on for me, I got an email from this friend who attended, yet thought I didn't want her to be there. I just don't understand how stuff like this happens in the midst of such a special moment. It was a crazy day and I tried to give my attention to each and every one of the individuals who were so kind in showing up. There is only one of me so I am sure that I wasn't able to give as much time as I wanted to each one. I was also very sick – despite the fact that I looked so healthy.

My email response to her was simple and straight-to-the-point, "Couldn't you tell how excited I was to see you?" I hadn't seen her in years and when I saw her at the event, I even offered to have lunch so we could have some one-on-one time. I am truly sorry she left feeling hurt like she did, but, you know, there is always someone that has themselves on their mind 24/7 and I wasn't going to let this steal my joy. I did the best I could to share myself with everyone who came out to show their support.

So, sometimes our Goliaths are external enemies and sometimes they are internal enemies - like our emotions. Emotional enemies are sometimes deep wounds of the heart and soul where we have been traumatized by someone - or something, along life's journey. Some call facing these emotional enemies *dealing with your demons* but, I prefer to call it *Facing Your Goliaths* (from one of my all-time favorite Bible stories).

1st Samuel, chapter 17 of the Bible tells the story of how David, as a young man, defeated Goliath - a 10 feet tall giant, using only three small stones and a slingshot. Not only did David not turn tail and run away, he bravely ran toward something much larger than himself and defeated the giant that stood there.

We all have giants to face in our lives. These *Goliaths* come in various shapes and sizes and include things like divorce, loss of a loved one, abuse that is sexual, emotional and/or physical in nature or, an array of other failures and disappointments. It is so much easier to run from the giants than to face them. But, avoidance only brings a false sense of peace and harmony. We think that *'ignorance is bliss'* but, in reality, not dealing with these *Goliaths* only ends up making both our emotional and physical self completely toxic. If thoughts generate 98% of disease, then 98% of all disease is avoidable. It is vital that you deal with what is eating at you on the inside.

When you are young and adored by everyone, it is easy to trust in people. After all, isn't that the great thing about being a child - your innocence? Unfortunately, there are people who have something dark inside them - their own

Goliath if you will. I believe that some of these kinds of people have a need to always control their environment or use those around them for their own desires - even at the expense of a child.

When I was in seventh grade, I was left alone with someone. I was around 12 or 13 at the time and still vividly remember every detail of what happened - even down to what I was wearing that day. All I need to say is that bad things were done to me that day. I will spare you – and me, the details because, even after all this time that has gone by, they are enough to make me extremely ill. As a young, frightened girl, I couldn't understand what had just happened to me and I honestly didn't know what to do.

I did go and tell another adult (one that I trusted) what had happened and I believe that this is what saved me from even more harm from this person in the ensuing years - even though this other adult never uttered a word in my defense. This other adult that I trusted enough to tell of this horrific incident did nothing but stand by in silence.

I still cannot comprehend why I was never comforted after what had happened and why I was left alone to deal with all of the emotions that I was feeling. This lack of action left me even more confused and hurt than ever because I now had to deal with the worst kind of betrayal from not one, but two adults that I trusted. One of them took horrible advantage of me and the other one stood by and did nothing.

I remember being sure of one thing and that was that I would *never* allow anyone to do that to me again. I know that a lot of young boys and girls who are victims of these very bad things are convinced that somehow *they* did something wrong or that *they* did something to deserve it, but, thankfully I never thought it was my fault and I knew absolutely - and without a doubt, that what had happened to me was wrong.

As I got older, this person's anger toward me escalated whenever we were together. I think that this individual believed they were under the microscope and that their behavior was being watched by others - even though no one had ever done anything to stop or report them. Or, it may just have been the guilt that was inside of them rearing its ugly head. Looking back on these things, it's hard not to feel a deep sense of sadness and betrayal from the *Dr. Jekyll & Mr. Hyde* personality that this person exhibited throughout my life.

Whenever I ran into them, I never knew if they were going to be fun, kind and encouraging or, the exact opposite. Although I mostly had times of normalcy - and even happy memories, in my life after that, I was never comfortable around this person and always walked on egg shells whenever I saw them. I was left feeling that I always had to try and gauge their emotional status. I truly believe that this person's guilt caused a Goliath to rise up in them.

I also honestly believe that this tragic event caused me to search for love in all the wrong places and in all the wrong ways. At the time, I didn't realize that I was in search of something but now, looking back, I am keenly aware of how my actions were affected by this event. By the time I was fifteen, I was partying hard. I finished high school while shoving most of these emotions deep down, filling my life with activities like playing volleyball, basketball and dreaming of my future.

After graduation, I moved across the country to California and became busy establishing myself as an Esthetician. I launched several new businesses, built friendships, fell in love and got married. After five years, my marriage came to a screeching halt and we divorced and went our separate ways.

During all of this time, it was nice to be on the opposite coast away from the scarred childhood memories that now lived only deep within my heart. I was also now in control of when I went to go and see everyone and I could stay for as long - or as short, of a time as I wanted to. The reality, though, was that I could not outrun this Goliath in my life.

As I had moved on with my life, I heard this person had become much more openly rude to others around him.

Prior to this point, he had been able to control his behavior in front of others. In fact, this individual was so good at hiding his dark side that no one would believe me when I would tell them that he had a problem. It was obvious to me that, one day soon, this giant secret was going to explode.

On rare occasions friends or family from my past would visit me in California and, one time, the woman who had walked away and failed to protect me when I asked for help came to see me. I was giving her a facial and talking about some of the horrible things that had happened to me - the things that had been swept under the rug and her response was, "Oh Venus, just let it go." She went on to say, "You'll be surprised at what you can let go." I then asked her what I wanted to ask her for years, "Why didn't anyone ever help me?" Her answer was "I told him if he ever hurt you again, I would call the police." I have to admit, it was nice to know that something actually had been done, but it certainly would have been nicer if I had been told that way back when it had happened. It would have been even nicer to know that someone validated my feelings and agreed with me that what had happened to me was very wrong.

I felt that if I had only been given the protection that I needed - and deserved, then this would have never happened. I felt if she had been there, then things would have been so different. I now saw that this person in

124

whom I put my trust and who I told what was going on, basically had a philosophy that ignoring something meant that it didn't happen. Maybe she honestly didn't know how to protect me and sometimes I still wonder if she was left to fend for herself as a child as well.

My *Goliath* was getting angrier and angrier and even more controlling, over the ensuing years and had gotten to the point that he had no problem ranting and raving in front of other people. Even when he was confronted by others about his verbally abusive behavior, it still continued.

During one visit, I saw these examples of what I had been hearing first hand and it took me a solid month to get over this trip. I became depressed and started struggling with all my horrid, haunting memories of childhood all over again. I knew that this Goliath was not going to go away.

During another trip a few years later, I saw him and was reminded again that some people try to do everything they can to control their environment - and the people in their lives, but now his Goliath was coming out of the closet and he was no longer able to control it. He had become quite offensive and would often say inappropriate things to others - especially women, even throwing frequent tantrums in public. As usual, there were also those who were close to him that continued to smile and behave as if nothing was wrong. They must have thought that if they were nice enough, others would overlook his horrid behavior.

I finally decided that I couldn't be around him anymore. Just dealing with his personality on infrequent phone calls had the ability to throw me into a full blown anxiety attack. Although he continued to try to get back into contact with me – mostly as an attempt to control me again, I didn't waiver on my decision. For the first time in my life, I started to feel in control.

So, I have set the stage of my battle against Goliath. Fast forward to when I am diagnosed with breast cancer and my head is spinning and all I can think of is how much I need support. Even though I let everyone in my life know that I am taking an alternative path for my healing - and that I am not be having surgery, chemo or radiation, I feel like they don't hear me. I feel like it goes in one ear and right out the other. Some simply don't believe me while others call to talk me out of it. While I understand their hesitation, they simply don't accept my decision to go on a path other than the traditional one for dealing with the cancer.

By this time, it has been a good five years since I have seen or spoken to the man who had taken advantage of me as a young girl. I sure wasn't ready to deal with 'all of that', especially now, because I am trying to keep my stress levels as low as possible in order to heal. God had other plans and knew that, in order to heal, I had to forgive.

So, during my journey of healing, I came to the realization that I did, in fact, have to face my Goliath. I know that it is time to take him on, all by myself - and defeat him. It is time to stop running from him. I know I have to figure out how to forgive him for what he has been done to me. You see, the pain that I experienced from what happened to me that day has caused me to be physically sick and I have never addressed it. I have only allowed it to eat away at me from the inside for all of these years. I knew this wasn't going to be easy but I wanted to be healthy again. No more running away.

Forgiveness doesn't just happen though, no matter how bad you want it to. It's a process. Sometimes it is a very long one and other times it is not so drawn out. For me, I had to work hard at even learning how to forgive. Slowly, as time went on, my heart was softening and I realized that I was beginning to forgive him. The uncomfortable feelings were slowly being replaced with compassion toward him. I am not saying I approve of what he did. This wasn't about him, it was about my reaction to what he did.

You may not understand why I forgave him and you may not believe that you can forgive the past hurts in your own life, but, the truth is, that the only person that you hurt when you don't forgive someone else is yourself.

The person who has hurt you has almost always moved on from the point of pain while you continue to stand in the midst of the hurt - even many years later. Forgiving someone else for their wrongs against you should be done for your own well being.

It brings about healing and restoration both physically and mentally. Remember that God has forgiven you for so much and, in the same manner; we are expected to forgive others - no matter how great the hurt. It doesn't mean that we say that the previous behavior is okay, it just means that we forgive and we move on and into a healthy state of mind.

It is also necessary in order to restore our relationship with God. Harboring unforgiveness is a sin and sin separates us from having a close relationship with our creator. Jesus, in teaching his disciples to pray said, "forgive us our sins _as_ we forgive those who sin against us." He then goes on to say in the very next sentence, "For if you do not forgive those who sin against you, neither will your Father in heaven forgive you your sins."

October 3rd, 2010 I was invited to a fitness retreat hosted by muscle activation specialist Teresa Tapp to speak on a topic that is near and dear to my heart - *"Is it* the Fear of the Disease?"   I am so excited to speak and share with others the wonderful things God has shown me on my journey.   I also know this is the time - and opportunity, that I need to face my Goliath, who is residing nearby to where the retreat is being held.

I know that if I want to be completely healed, I have to face my giant.   I have absolutely no fear or anxiety in going to visit this time around.   Finding out that I am going, some who know me are very uptight about it all while others are living in the land of denial - the place where everything is fine and nothing could ever go wrong. You know, telling me to "just keep smiling and everything will be OK."

As for me?   I am glad to see everyone and, for some reason, I laugh and enjoy the whole time I am there. *"Therefore my heart is glad and my glory (my inner self) rejoices; my body too shall rest and confidently dwell in safety."* - Psalm 16:9   For the first time in my life, this person's behavior didn't bother me at all.   God had enabled me to change my thoughts and the way that I felt toward him. He had miraculously made it possible for me to truly forgive him so that I could find peace within myself and not be affected by his behavior anymore.

When we were leaving, a friend told me that I had handled the situation so much better than they would have.   I was able to share with her that this was all God's doing and how He had changed me so that I could come out on the other side of the fire strong and whole. *"I can do all things through Christ who strengthens me."* - Philippians 4:13

Since the breast cancer was diagnosed, I did several different detox programs in order to rid my body of toxins. By now I felt – and knew, that my body was pretty clean although, for some reason, I decided to do another six-week detox. During this particular detox for my colon, kidneys, liver, gallbladder and my blood, I found myself much more easily agitated and easily angered. I am usually 'full of life' and a very 'happy-go-lucky' person, so anger is not the norm for me. Little did I know that God was using this particular detox to bring about a complete spiritual detox as well.

A few weeks later, the woman I had counted on to defend me from my Goliath and who I had asked for help, called me. I told her that I still didn't understand why she hadn't stood up for me when I was a child when I had told her I needed help. (I know she had told me she had threatened him to call the police if he ever did it again, yet I didn't feel that was good enough). She was crying - just asking for forgiveness over and over, stating that she just didn't have enough self esteem to stand up to him for me.

At that moment, I had an epiphany. I realized for the first time that I had built up even more anger against her than the person who had done such horrible things to me. I expressed to her how angry I was and how I felt that she hadn't stood up for me all those years ago. I told her that children *must* be put first and taken care of no matter what.

The next day, I was trying to use my copier at work and it didn't do what I wanted it to do. All of a sudden something snapped in me and all the years of bottled up anger at this person (who left me to fend for myself) took over. I slammed the copier on the floor, jumped up and down on it, beat it and threw it against the wall. I tore that copier to pieces so bad that my poor dog ran and hid because he had never seen me behave like this. I then ran outside, with pieces of the copier, and threw them on the front lawn.

I didn't even know that I was strong enough to do the damage that I did but, when it was all said and done, I felt like the weight of the world had been lifted off my shoulders. My friends still joke about the copier saying that it was like a scene from the TV sitcom *The Office*. I always seem to do these strange, crazy things in moments of stress in my life.

The next day, all my dog walker could talk about was how smashed up the copier was on the front lawn. He was amazed that it was so mangled and said that it looked like someone had thrown it from the top floor of the apartment building. He went on to say that the weirdest thing about it was that my dog insisted on walking over and peeing on it. I laughed so hard, I almost cried as I told him that it was my copier and that my dog was apparently saying, "Piss on you copier for making my mom so mad!"

So, when everything was said and done, I realized, after all these years, that my actual Goliath not only who I originally thought but also the person I had asked for help and who I felt should have protected me. In fact, I felt she was the larger Goliath because she never stood up for or protected me. I now saw that my anger towards her was more intense. Some of my feelings were coming from the fact that I knew that the person who had hurt me had probably been mentally ill. Although she had no idea he would ever violate me or that I was in harm's way the day I was left alone with him, I still partially blamed her.

God had helped me find a way to forgive him and now I needed His help again in finding a way to forgive her. I started this process by reciting forgiveness affirmations every day. I would say "I forgive you, I love you and I bless you." This may sound corny to you but this is what I really did and, you know what? After saying something repeatedly it actually becomes the truth and I was able to forgive her.

In order to defeat your own *Goliaths*, you must figure out what the issues of *your* heart are and what's really eating at you on the inside. We all have areas of unforgiveness in our lives. In order to heal emotionally and physically, you need to address these wounds that you have buried away deep within yourself.

When I interview women who have come to me for help in healing their breast cancer, the first question I ask them is, "What do you think the root cause of your diagnosis is?" The number one response I get is, "Stress."

The most interesting discovery that I keep finding when I uncover the deep issues of the heart with these women is that most of them have experienced a bad relationship - or that there is someone who has hurt them deeply that they have never been able to forgive.

Any painful experience can create a lack of trust and, according to Dr. Alex Lloyd, author of the bestselling book *The Healing Code*, breast cancer is a trust and patience issue. Trust is the absolute biggest issue that has to be dealt with when it comes to breast cancer.

As for me, I believe that breast cancer is also a matter of the heart. Think about it. The breasts are just above where your heart lies. You feed your children from your breasts. When your children hurt themselves, you lay their head against them and you stroke their back and tell them that everything is going to be okay. Everything about the breast area of your body has to do with nurturing. A broken heart – or broken trust, can definitely lead to physical and emotional disease.

You will never heal unless you defeat your own Goliath. Remember, it is faster and easier to go *through* the mountain than to take the long way around it. In order to heal physically, you must get to the emotional root of your problems.

Dr. Caroline Leaf, author of the program *Switch On Your Brain with a 5-Step Learning Process,* says, "Every gene lies dormant until a thought activates it." My breast (the one with cancer in it) didn't cause the cancer, so cutting one (or both) of them off just wasn't logical to me. I had to determine what thoughts I had experienced in the recent or distant past that would cause cancer to grow in my breast. Praying and truly seeking this answer, I found that my inability or unwillingness to forgive certain people was definitely one of, if not '*the*' root(s) of my problem.

In addition to the repressed memories in our minds, we *have* to deal with what Dr. Leaf refers to as cell memory. Every trauma we have in our life – whether physical or emotional - affects our cells and our cells have memory. For example, I didn't even realize that much of my anger was directed at a completely different person than I originally thought. In fact, she was a person that always seemed like a victim herself so this brought out my own protective instincts, making me feel sorry for her.

I thought I had to protect her instead of realizing that, as an adult, it was *her* job to protect me - the child. Once I finally figured out what was eating on me from the inside - and addressed it, I was able to begin building healthy relationships with them and accepting them for who they are. I also had a brand new foundation to build healthy relationships with others. It is so refreshing to be able to relate to everyone without putting unrealistic expectations on them and to live a life that is free of unforgiveness – even if that unforgiveness is buried so deep you don't know it is there.

God not only allowed me to find the unforgiveness buried in my heart and mind, He also granted me the compassion and grace to forgive those who hurt me. This process has proven to me that forgiveness must be given to those who wrong us in order for us to heal ourselves and promote our own well-being. And, I learned it is equally important to forgive ourselves. Often we cannot truly accept God's forgiveness - or the forgiveness of others, when it is extended. So, give and receive forgiveness freely.

The good news is that there are many tools available to assist you when dealing with your own emotional and physical *Goliaths*. I recommend prayer, devotional time, finding a local church that can help support you emotionally and seeing a good counselor that can properly direct you. I also recommend reading *The Healing Code*. If done consistently and properly you will find great peace in utilizing these 'codes'.

Just remember, you can't just cut, poison or burn yourself to solve the root of your problem. This only gets rid of the physical manifestation of the problem, not the problem itself. On top of that, the physical manifestation often just comes roaring back. Most individuals - and their doctors, treat only the symptom - which is the cancer. So, even if you choose the best natural or the best conventional plan for treatment and fail to address the root problem, the symptom (cancer) will just resurface again and again.

"Trust in the Lord with all your heart, and do not lean on your own understanding; in all your ways acknowledge Him and He will make your paths straight." - Proverbs 3:5-6 ask God to show you the truth and to give you the wisdom and ability to work through your problems. Learn to trust again, starting with God because He is the only one who will never fail you.

The truth will set you free. God's word says that in Him and knowing Him is freedom - and it was for the freedom of our souls that Jesus died. The whole purpose of defeating your *Goliath* is so that God's healing balm will cure the sickness of the soul and let you live the most abundant life He has planned for you.

Then said David to Goliath, "You come to me with a sword, a spear and a javelin, but I come to you in the name of the Lord." - 1st Samuel 17:45 just like David, with God on your side, you *can* defeat your own *Goliath*.

It is very important to me to close out this chapter with a warning to all adults about the importance of protecting children from harm. It is the adults' absolute responsibility to do everything to prevent harm and to address any concerns or situations any child brings to their attention. Don't ignore or minimize any problem and think it will go away. You must investigate any incidents thoroughly and take them seriously. God gave us stewardship over children to raise them in a healthy and secure environment.

I can now close this chapter of my life no longer running away from the giants in my life for my *Goliath* has been defeated.

A letter is an important way to say what you want to say - whether you end up giving it to the person or burning it ceremonially. Either way, you are getting rid of the toxic effect on your body by saying it out loud. Although I kept mine short and sweet, you can use it as a template – (expanding and/or changing it as needed for your own letter). Here is the letter that I sent.

Dear ---------,

I send you this letter to remind you and make sure that you know that I have forgiven you for everything you have done in the past. Though there were difficult times that we went through, I do recognize and see the good parts of you too. Now it's time for you to ask God for forgiveness and to forgive yourself.

Love,

Venus

"You God, are a healing balm and your grace is a medicine that we can apply to our hearts that brings forth spiritual and emotional healing."

- Lisa Smith

"For if you forgive others their sins, your heavenly Father will also forgive you, but, if you do not forgive others their sins, neither will your Father forgive your sins."

- Jesus, in Matthew 6:14-15

Is It the Fear or the Disease?

Cancer. Just saying the word can create fear in a person's heart. People immediately think of the worst-case scenario when this word is spoken over them.

When an individual, who is diagnosed with any type of cancer, has the difficult task of informing friends and family, the automatic reaction they receive is one of compassion and sorrow. Staring face to face with those they love, fear also exudes immediately from their eyes. Yes, FEAR (that four letter word), quickly overtakes them. You wonder, is the fear in their eyes primarily because they are praying that they will never get it? Cancer is not contagious but the fear is. We put so much of our hope, when it comes to cancer and other diseases, in so-called special interest groups and non-profits to finally develop a cure. It seems that all we get in exchange for putting our hope in them is another year of empty promises.

One question stirs deeply within me when I see so many people participating in these 'pink' events. How many more walks do they think they have to attend and how many more pink ribbon products do they think they have to buy before there's a cure? I believe that women in the 'pink club' secretly think that if they exhaustively invest their efforts in working hard to raise money for a cure, they will somehow earn extra 'karma points' that they can cash in if they are ever diagnosed. Sometimes I get the feeling that they are working so hard on 'pink' causes because of the fear that they will be the next one diagnosed, hoping their efforts will find a cure by then.

All this pink, yet NO CURE! Please don't misunderstand me; I honestly do get why so much energy and effort is put into these causes. I know it's primarily because women are extremely compassionate and sympathetic and that they truly want to help. And yes, they want to find a cure. Don't we all? I also know that cancer is big business.

Have a look at this article that refers to some of the excesses discovered by the *The Cancer Letter* (a watch-dog over the world of cancer care) at the very same Disneyland of Cancer that I went to (you just can't make this stuff up),

The financially stressed cancer center in Texas seems to have invested at least $1.5 million in a new 'corporate' office suite that will be home to the wife of the cancer center's president. These revelations come in an article published today in *The Cancer Letter*.

The Cancer Letter used the Texas Public Information Act to obtain 680 pages of documents that describe the project as an "Office Renovation". However, the article argues, a renovation it was not. The 25,000-square-foot suite is located on the sixth floor of the just-constructed south campus research building.

The cancer center president's wife moved to Texas when her husband became president in 2011. She was hired as the scientific director of the new drug-discovery center and as the chair of the cancer center's department of genomic medicine which aims to enlist drug companies in promising collaborations.

Among the itemized expenses reported in *The Cancer Letter* are nearly $28,000 for settees, lounge chairs and reception area tables as well as about $210,000 for translucent walls. The spending on the walls was thought to be so extravagant that it required a variance - or special permission, from the university's executive vice-chancellor for health affairs.

The cancer center defended its actions saying it raised $15 million in donations from private individuals. They said that the existing space was not configured to support their new concept and that the "re-designed" space would "create an open environment of communication, provide an appropriate meeting space for high-level industry decision-makers and support a new suite in computational biology."

This is not the first time that the cancer center's wife has landed in the public spotlight since she arrived at the huge, high-profile cancer center in Texas. Last year, there was an outcry after her research team was awarded an $18-million grant from the Cancer Prevention and Research Institute of Texas (CPRIT) because her grant bypassed the scientific peer review process in obtaining the funds.

All of this while her husband, the president of the cancer center, was announcing austerity measures such as suspension of merit raises and slowing of hiring for all of its employees. Here is an excerpt from an email sent to the cancer center's employees,

"For most of the last year, our operating expense have exceeded our operating revenue (meaning that we've spent more than we've made from providing our patient care services). What we're facing today is much like what you'd face with your own checkbook if you had spent more than you were paid for several months."

I certainly hope that, after reading my book, someone will be inspired to start working passionately to promote any non-profit organizations that generously give to those who wish to choose the natural route. Most individuals do not have the financial means to do so. You may not be fully aware of the fact that insurance companies do not cover most, if any, alternative treatments. They only pay for conventional treatments.

This is, in large part, due to the fact that no one is going to fund scientific research that looks at the healing benefits of natural treatments because there is no money in it for the medical community. Imagine how much money would be lost for hospitals, doctors, pharmacies, and pharmaceutical companies if individuals chose to let their body heal itself naturally.

Almost all individuals diagnosed with cancer choose the conventional method not just because of fear, but also due to that fact that their insurance will only pay for burning, cutting and poisoning them. It's a crazy world.

I am working diligently to establish a non-profit organization that will assist those who have been diagnosed with cancer. I also hope it will help those who want to make preventative lifestyle changes in regards to their health. I have learned so much on this journey and I refuse to sit back, timidly, and watch others be overtaken by fear or barbaric methods of 'treatment'. I want to share the wealth of knowledge I have gained because they – and you, deserve to know the truth – THERE ARE OTHER OPTIONS.

So, don't let fear drive your decisions. Did you know that, when a person is delivered a diagnosis - or told that there is a chance they may have cancer, their cortisol levels rise so high that the adrenals burn out and *that* can put the body into death mode. *"For God has not given us a spirit of fear but, rather instead, one of power and of love and of a sound mind."* - 2 Timothy 1:7

I have asked myself the question, "Why do we look at cancer the way we do?" Think about it for a moment. Much of what we know about cancer has been carefully put together by the pharmaceutical industry and their media propaganda. Ever see an ad on TV for a drug. Ask yourself, "If their drugs are so good, then why do they have to advertise?" Congress even recently passed legislation to limit the influence of drug reps on doctors, trying to prevent such abuses as offering financial incentives – including trips, for writing prescriptions.

Doctors and pharmaceutical companies may not purposely intend to keep us in the dark about the amazing superiority of using natural methods to heal cancer, but they sure don't have a profit-incentive to promote it. Money is the main reason why detailed studies are not being done on natural methods. Not many research labs are going to do double-blind, controlled studies on any natural methods of healing because they will have no way to recoup their investment and no real way to develop a patented, marketable drug.

Most individuals, who are diagnosed with cancer knee-jerk out of fear and, within days, agree to let doctors set up an expensive 'treatment' regimen which often includes chemo, radiation or surgery (and sometimes all three). Can you blame them? It is not easy to stand up to a doctor who has gone to school for umpteen years. It can be intimidating to challenge their knowledge – and they don't make it easy either. After paying well over $100,000 for their education – often in the form of looming student loans, doctors often act arrogant or offended if you challenge their knowledge. It is the fear that they know something that you don't that leads to choosing expensive 'treatment' methods that often simply do not work. So, if knowledge keeps individuals from reacting out of fear and mis-information, then what exactly is cancer?

Well, to begin with, it's a multi-billion-dollar business! I'm here to tell you, cancer as a money-maker is alive and well on planet earth. Did you know that, depending on the individual case and the type (and number) of treatments needed, the total cost of breast cancer treatment, on average, can run $100,000 or, in advanced cases, $300,000? And that's an average. There have been cases where women with breast cancer were billed as much as $500,000 or even $1 million dollars for their medical expenses.

Even with the billions of dollars that are poured into research a year, western medicine has only improved cancer survival rates by only 2.3% to 5% In the last 55 years. These startling statistics should stir you to be proactive in your health, creating a desire within you to develop good habits that can prevent cancer. One In five of us will be diagnosed with it in our lifetime. Don't wait to get started with a prevention plan.

How about looking at it from this perspective, if 2,600 woman get breast cancer and they all choose the currently accepted 'normal' or 'conventional' route of chemo, surgery and possibly radiation, five years later only 36 of these women will still be alive. Let me leave this little nugget for your to ponder upon as well, "There is no cure for chemo!" Chemo, if you live through it, does damage to the body that no medical science can repair. So, the choice is yours today, do you want sit idly by, waiting for a cure or do you want to be a pioneer and help your body heal itself?

If you have not yet been diagnosed with cancer, I believe that prevention is the only sensible thing for a person to do. If you do have cancer, I believe the overall plan I have outlined in this book is your best option. Think about it, you are reading a book written by someone who chose not to have chemo or radiation or surgery. My doctors and health care providers made me feel like I had to follow their plan and that there were no other options.

There are, in fact, many doctors who offer alternative cancer treatments. These physicians are forced to treat their patients outside of the United States because the alternative treatment is considered illegal here in the U.S. by the FDA. What a crying shame that, in the land of the free, we are not allowed to choose our own methods of medical treatment.

What if we look at cancer in a different light? If it is a biological process that requires certain conditions for the process to initiate (and tumors are the symptoms and products of this process), then cancer is not the actual tumor itself, but, instead, it is the process that is producing the tumor. To clarify, let's look at the tumor as a symptom of the underlying problem rather than as the actual underlying problem itself.

If this is the case, then by the time the tumor is seen, felt or diagnosed, you have may have had 'cancer' for years – maybe even decades. The most important thing to do - even before ever being diagnosed, is to shut down the process that leads to tumors or cancers of any type.

People are fooled into thinking that if they cut, burn or poison their body, the process will be shut down. This is not the case. These methods only attempt to eradicate the end result of the process. Conventional treatment only takes care of the symptoms, not the cause, leaving a vast opportunity for the cancer to return even stronger the second time around.

Statistically, if the same expensive clinical trial studies were done for natural methods that are done for pharmaceutical drugs, I believe the results would be startling. It may show that those cancer patients who avoid orthodox medicine and go the alternative route might actually live longer lives or achieve higher cure rates.

The medical community has even become afraid to use the word 'cure'. It is considered bad practice to ever use it. Why? Is it because they are afraid of giving false hope? No. It is mainly because they know that the cancer still lurks somewhere inside of your body. They know that they have not stopped the process, but, instead, that they have only fought back the symptoms.

If those who choose the natural route stay consistent with their preventative health measures - and continue to do their homework along the way, they will reap the healthy benefits of their due diligence and may end up cancer-free. While the medical community at large sees anything other than chemo, radiation and surgery as a gamble, I will take those odds any day over 2.3 to 5% survival rates of conventional methods.

Chemo not only severely damages the body, but, those who fall prey to putting their hope in it will more than likely see their cancer return down the road. It will also often be stronger and more violent than before. I talk to individuals all of the time that have experienced this to be true. I believe it is primarily due to the fact that the doctors are not addressing the underlying process – not to mention how badly chemo and radiation overload and weaken the immune system.

I just met a woman recently, who had been diagnosed with stage-one breast cancer and she chose the conventional route. After going through surgery and chemo, she was then given a clean bill of health - for a short period of time. Upon returning to her doctor for a checkup, she was informed that the cancer had returned with a vengeance and had now spread to her liver, her lymphatic system and was now stage-four cancer.

Guess what she chose to do? She went back for more! More burning, more poison, and hopeless promises from her doctors. I really shouldn't say that she 'chose' to go back for more. What other options did she have? They sure weren't offering any alternatives. Who knows? Maybe this time it will cure her. I doubt it. The main goal of this book is to let you know that there are other options and that you can overcome the fear that surrounds you when making the best choices for your own healing or prevention plan.

My hope and prayer is that these statistics will alarm you more than the fear that you become consumed with when you are diagnosed. Instead of letting it grip you, allow the fear to drive you down a healthy path of healing. Turn your fear into a walk of faith. Choose the only option that addresses the process instead of just the symptoms.

Why are people so convinced that conventional treatments are the only way to go? Here are some of the reasons I think people choose the way they do:

- Medical Professionals are addicted to using drugs to cure a symptom (in this case cancer) instead of stopping the underlying process or finding ways of prevention. Individuals with cancer themselves contribute to the problem. They feel that if there were a real cure for their cancer, then their doctor would know about it. So, they assume a cure doesn't exist and that the prescribed maintenance program is their best option. They fail to research all of the other options available to them. Instead of having faith in their own ability to make choices that will let their bodies heal the way God designed them to, they instead let their doctors becomes their god.

- Medical professionals are addicted to the idea that they are the only qualified ones with answers. This is not the case. This book is not a condemnation of the talented individuals who fill the health-care system. It is a wake-up call. While I respect the many years of learning that conventional doctors, physician assistants, nurses and medical technicians have invested, some things have to dramatically change if individuals are going to survive and thrive after being diagnosed with cancer and other diseases. I have met some amazing holistic doctors who offer alternative treatments and I have also met some conventional doctors who have made significant changes to the way they treat their patients. They see the same problems I do and have discovered the truth when it comes to comparing their old methods vs. the natural ways of treating disease.

- Once again it comes back to money! The

pharmaceutical companies want patients (consumers) to try and cure themselves through medication, not prevention and holistic treatments because every person who gets cancer increases their shareholders' value. You won't see a pharmaceutical company encouraging a doctor to do anything other than to prescribe their drug.

- Does this sound harsh? I hope so! Maybe somehow by reading this book it will open your eyes, mind and heart and help you to get proactive about your own personal cancer treatment and health prevention plan.

If all disease is a biological process that has a definite point of origin, then it can most likely be halted. In other words, if it can be turned on, then it can be turned off. Even better is that, because the body can heal itself, it can not only be turned off, the damage can also often be repaired and the process reversed.

We should be looking at the disease process from a different angle. From my own personal experience - and all of the research I have done, I believe that diseases (or health issues in general) are, in large part, due to malfunctioning, oxygen-depleted cells.

There are many pathways to becoming imbalanced. Dr

Andreas Moritz believes that cancer is a survival mechanism of the body. He says that it is the body saying, "Stop with all the bad habits, I'm on toxic overload, it's time to turn the switch off." But, most of us want a magic little pill instead of changing our lifestyles. That always amazes me because I truly want to live my life and live it to the fullest. If only everyone would do their homework and learn how beneficial eating and living healthy is, how eye opening would that be?

Ann Wigmore, known as "the mother of living foods", was an early pioneer in the use of wheatgrass juice and living foods for detoxifying and healing the body, mind, and spirit. I like to say she was in the 'health field' as opposed to what I refer to as the 'death field'. In the health field, the emphasis is on prevention and restoring the body to a healthy state once disease sets in. She and others in this field believe that deficiencies and toxemia are the main causes of all disease.

So, cleanse the body, the mind and the spirit and the body will heal itself. We must never forget that, in the not so distant past - before the 1940's, we were a much healthier people. Our food was real and we didn't consume large amounts of sugar and junk food as we do today. There were also fewer pesticides, dyes, chemicals, drug therapies and there were definitely no genetically modified (GMO) foods like we have today.

People were much more connected, they moved their bodies more and they valued God, country and family to a higher degree than we see today. Today, we live such fast paced lives, always on the go, eating on the go, always connected to some kind of technical device and we are no longer paying attention to what's most important. No wonder cancer, heart disease and obesity are at epidemic proportions!

I want to remind you of the most important thing of all, God almighty created our bodies and He does all things perfectly. We are meant to function in wholeness and perfect health just the way we were created. I believe one day in the future people will look back on how cancer was treated and think "how barbaric" just the way we now look at how bloodletting was used in the late 18th century.

I am going to say it again, "Prevention is the key!" Stand up for your rights to have organic real food, not the genetically modified foods which are being sold in our supermarkets. While it may make food cheaper for us or more profitable for those who grow or sell it, I beg of you to say "No!" to this monstrosity of "Frankenfoods'.

Let me close with this thought once again for you to really ponder ... "Is it the fear or the disease"?

What's driving you to make the decisions you are making concerning your health? The fear of a health crisis should drive you to making healthy lifestyle changes. The fear of conventional methods should drive you to stay away from treatments that break your body down.

Remember to pause first. Get away if you can. Remove the fear. Remove yourself from those around you who are fearful. Pray and seek God for wisdom concerning your health, then apply His wisdom in making the right decisions concerning your entire well-being.

"For wisdom is a defense even as money is a defense, but the excellence of knowledge is that wisdom shields and preserves the life of him who has it." - *Ecclesiastes 7:11-13*

Let knowledge and wisdom be the key to your health success. Replace fear with blind faith, I am living proof that it will lead you to a path of healing and wholeness.

Delight yourself in the Lord and he will give you the desires of your heart. - *Psalm 37:4*

Remarkable Path

Remarkable: re·mark·a·ble - to be worthy of notice or commenting on, worthy of attention, striking. Synonyms: extraordinary, exceptional, amazing, astonishing, astounding, marvelous, wonderful, sensational, stunning, incredible, unbelievable, phenomenal, outstanding, momentous. When I think back on the journey I have been on for the last couple of years, the word remarkable comes to mind - and all of its synonyms. It truly has been full of incredible – and sometime intense, moments. It has also been filled with God's love and direction. I am so thankful for the existing friendships and new relationships that have enhanced each and every day during this period of my life. I wish I could share every experience with you. This book is just some of the highlights that I thought you would enjoy reading about.

Remarkable Relationships.

The relationships I have had in the past couple of years are filled with connections that put me in touch with critical people who had valuable knowledge and expertise that I could apply to my health. Some of these relationships were also cultivated into friendships that I will cherish for a lifetime. Networking and connections indeed prove to be powerful tools. One call led to another, then to another... What an array of wonderful people!

Dr. Hines, for example, is an intelligent and caring physician who imparted a wealth of information to me pertaining to my health. I am so grateful to have met him and I always enjoyed contacting his office, often talking to his wife. During one of our conversations, she provided me with a contact she thought would be beneficial to me. She told me about Michelle Hart, who owns a

Thermography company called DITI Imaging (www.ditiimaging.com). I contacted Michelle and gathered details from her regarding her company and shared my story with her. During our conversation, she told me about a dear friend of hers, Chris Templeton, who once was an actress on the well-known soap, *The Young and the Restless.*

From a young age, Chris suffered from polio, yet overcame all obstacles and was one of the first successful handicapped actresses. At the time I spoke with Michelle, Chris had been battling cancer for close to ten years. She introduced us and Chris was so warm and caring, making it easy for our friendship to quickly blossom. I stayed in touch with her on the phone and, during one of our chats; she shared her own personal health struggles as well as her passion to help others in need. Her compassion for those fighting cancer inspired her to start a foundation called RAWtatoilli. The primary goal of RAWtatolll was to deliver raw food to cancer patients. Now that's remarkable!

One day I decided that I wanted to meet this lovely lady in person so I took a trip to down to San Antonio - only a hop, skip and a jump from Austin. While I was there, she shared with me her plans to travel over all of U.S. in search of treatments that would cure her. We were always one another's cheerleader, rooting for each other to be healed and healthy once again.

The pressure and stress seemed too much for her most of the time as she continued her search for treatments that might improve her health. In an effort to do something special for her, I decided to donate ten percent of the proceeds from the fundraiser my friends threw for me. I knew this would allow her to receive some special IV treatments that she really wanted. Unfortunately, her health took a downhill spiral and she's now cheering me - and her loved-ones, on as she smiles down from heaven pain-free, healed and whole.

Fast forward several months and one day at my office, I was reviewing a consultation sheet from one of my clients. She indicated that she regularly did something called a T-Tapp workout. Curious, I asked her what it was. She explained that T-Tapp is a nuerokentic compound-muscle workout, mainly targeting the lymphatic system. This triggered an interest within me to learn more because of the line of work that I am in as an Esthetician. Later, when I had a chance, I did some additional research on Teresa Tapp's website to learn more about this routine and her products. Another remarkable connection made!

The information I found out about this lymphatic workout was fascinating and enlightening. I ordered several of her beginner videos and I still, to this very day, enjoy doing the T-Tapp workout. I highly recommend that you take some time to familiarize yourself with Teresa and the amazing tools and workshops she offers. (www.t-tapp.com).

Teresa Tapp is beautiful, inspiring, intelligent, full of life and her energy has certainly blessed me beyond words. One day I received an email from her inviting me to share my speech *"Is It the Fear or the Disease"* at one of her beauty boot camps (as I mentioned earlier in the book). I gladly accepted her invitation and I can't express how excited I was to get this golden opportunity. I had no earthly idea if I would be a good public speaker or not. The only thing I knew for sure was that God had given me this chance to share a message with others that could change their lives. He chose me for this particular time! What a privilege and honor that He trusts me that much.

October 22nd, 2010 The time has finally arrived for me to hop on a plane and head to Florida to speak at the beauty boot camp. Not only am I thrilled about my speaking engagement, but my sister and her best friend are joining me at the event. What an adrenaline rush! I love every single minute of it! It's my first time giving my speech to a crowd.

The feedback I received was so amazing and encouraged me so much! A brand new beginning and I knew that this was exactly what I wanted to do. I wanted to inspire others to take care of themselves, to be proactive with their health and prevent disease by sharing my story and the wealth of information I had obtained along my remarkable path.

After the retreat concluded, we are all gathered in the bar area downstairs at the hotel. Let me set the stage for you before I go any further. A few months prior to this speaking engagement, I was watching Sid Roth, the host of a show called *It's Supernatural* (www.sidroth.org). On this particular show, his guest was a pastor by the name of Billy Burke. Pastor Billy shared how he was healed of cancer by Kathryn Kuhlman. As a young man, he had been diagnosed with brain cancer and was given only three weeks to live. His grandmother, who knew the Great Physician (God) could do anything, decided to take him to a service where Kathryn Kuhlman was ministering. That evening, Kathryn laid hands on him and he was immediately healed. That miraculous event changed his life forever. From that time on, Pastor Billy continued to study under Kathryn leadership until she passed away. He now travels worldwide preaching about God's grace and His healing power.

The Remarkable Healer!

If you are not familiar with the Bible, I hope you will take some time to read it and also to research the information I am sharing with you. *"Jesus went throughout Galilee, teaching in their synagogues, preaching the good news of the kingdom and healing every disease and sickness* among the people." - Matthew 4:23 you may ask, "Does Jesus still heal today?" The answer to your question is, "Yes! He does." *"Jesus Christ is the same yesterday, today and forever." - Hebrews 13:8 His* healing touch still applies to us as much today as it did when He was walking the earth.

I was completely mesmerized by Sid Roth's show and Pastor Billy Burke's testimony of how God healed him. I immediately went online to gather more details about his ministry. To my surprise, it is located in Tampa, Florida - just twenty minutes from where I would be speaking. I decided to attend one of his services while I was in Florida and I wondered if I would have the opportunity to actually meet him.

I love how God directs our footsteps. There we were, gathering in the bar area of the hotel with the featured speakers and all of those who put the amazing boot camp together. As I enter into the bar, I sat down next to a lady named Shelly Ballestero who also spoke at the event, (www.beautybygodbook.com). She immediately said to me, "You're the real thing."

As we talked about the event, she then asked if I would, by chance, be interested in meeting Pastor Billy Burke? Keep in mind that I had said nothing to her about Pastor Billy nor did I even know that she knew him. I asked her, "How do you know Billy Burke"? She told me that her husband was the head worship leader for his ministry. Coincidence? Not at all! It was our remarkable God.

I excitedly told her that I had just watched him on a segment of the Sid Roth show. We quickly made plans to meet Saturday night and attend one of his services. I was so excited that I told an older couple from Minnesota who I met shortly afterwards all about it. They too were big fans of his and asked if they could join us.

October 24th, 2010 Saturday night is finally here. As we are driving to the church that evening, I had these preconceived ideas, thinking he must pastor a huge church since he travels constantly speaking to thousands. But, in actuality, he ministers to a local church of approximately 100 people. Instead of a traditional building, they have their church service in a large meeting room at the Marriott hotel. It was not what I expected, but, miracles can happen anywhere. After all, Jesus was always en-route to somewhere when he encountered individuals in need of a healing touch.

As we entered into the room, my new friend Shelly took us directly to the front row where her husband Angelo had reserved seating for us. As the service began, it was a bit different and on a smaller scale than what I was used to. There were no tele-prompters, the band was smaller and they sang a lot of the older hymns – most of which I did not know. The older couple from Minnesota who came with us – Sam and Abigail, knew all the songs and words. I didn't care, every time I heard the word Jesus, I would raise my hand and say, "Jesus!" It didn't stop me from thoroughly enjoying myself.

We had the best seats in house. Pastor Billy was right in front of us. He's such a dynamic preacher! As he concluded his message, he looked over at Sam and Abigail and asked them to stand up and invited them toward him. As they stood there, Pastor Billy prayed for Sam first, barely touching his forehead, and Sam hits the floor, slain in the Spirit. Pastor Billy then prays for Abigail and the same thing happens to her. The presence of God was so strong in the room that night!

Suddenly, I hear Shelly's husband, Angelo, say, "Get over here and have him pray for you." Sam and Abigail are now coming back to their senses and return to their seats. Pastor Billy continues to overlook me as he is praying for others. He finally walks over to me and, as I am standing there in my dress, I turn to the man who comes up behind me that I call a "catcher" and say, "Whatever happens, don't let my dress fly up." This man's job was to make sure that no one hurt themselves as they fall.

Pastor Billy is standing right in front of me and asks, "What do you need God to do in your life?" I tell him about the large tumor in my breast and he asks me what stage of breast cancer it is. I tell him it doesn't matter, I just want it gone and that it is time for this to be over! He begins to pray over me and lightly touches my forehead and down I go to the floor!

Thank God Abigail came over and covered my legs with her husband's jacket. He proceeds to tell me to stay on the floor and, while I am lying there, he begins to ask the crowd who knows me. Sam and Abigail say, "She's with us". He asks them my name and they tell him, "Venus, her name is Venus!" Pastor Billy looks down at me and says these very powerful and anointed words as he gave me a word of knowledge by the Holy Spirit, "Venus, no knife will every touch your body, be healed, whether you think you deserve it or you don't believe you deserve it - you are healed."

He told me to touch my breast and when I did, what I felt was astonishing. What was once a large mass was now a very small lump. Praise God for His remarkable touch!

When I returned to my seat, I was so full of gratitude that I just kept crying and hugging Abigail. As the time of ministry and prayer continues, I decide to step out to the restroom to freshen up. As I was heading toward the door, I saw Pastor Billy praying over a woman who gave her name as Glenda. She was a beautiful lady with long black hair. As he was talking to her, she told him that she had stage-four cancer. A few minutes later, as I came back into the room, Glenda was walking down the aisle to return to her seat so I paused for a moment to give her a hug, never saying a word to her.

At this point, Pastor Billy is going around the room, touching all of the people on the forehead and I was not going to let him forget about me! Even though he already said that I was healed, I started saying, "Me, me, me next, me next." I am not sure what Pastor Billy must have thought of me and I didn't care, the presence of God was so strong that I wanted all I could get.

You may be quite skeptical right now and wonder what it means to be "slain in the Spirit." To be slain in the Spirit you first have to be willing to yield to the Holy Spirit of God. As you stand waiting to be prayed for, you turn your thoughts toward how good God is and how He gave His all for us by sending His Son Jesus to the cross so that we might be made whole.

Being slain in the Spirit is simply when the presence and power of God comes onto you so strongly that it causes you to either fall forward or backward. His power can either come directly through the hands of someone operating under the Lord's anointing or directly on you by God Himself, such as when you see people falling to the ground while just sitting in their seats with no one laying a hand on them. *"Then He brought me by way of the north gate to the front of the temple so I looked and behold, the glory of the Lord filled the house of the Lord and **I fell on***

my face." - *Ezekiel 44:4*

God is God. He can move and operate in whatever fashion He feels is necessary to bless us and heal us. I refuse to limit Him nor will I doubt what He is capable of doing. He is Creator, He is Savior, and He is our remarkable God.

It was so surreal when we left and returned to our hotel. I wrote down the words that were spoken over me that night to keep them as a reminder of the hope and encouragement I received. I normally do not sleep well in hotels because of things like mold or dander in the rugs, bedding or the air conditioning system but, that night, the peace of God was hovering over me and I slept like a baby. What a remarkable experience!

The next day, when I was checking out of the hotel, I ran into Glenda and her husband (who was sporting several large crosses around his neck). She turned to her husband and said "Honey, this is the lady I was telling you about from last night." What had happened to me during the service obviously affected others that were there that evening. We formally introduced ourselves and she said, "Look what the chemo is doing to me – it's just brutal."

As she and I were talking, her husband excitedly shared that he too had a healing ministry. He went on to tell me that they both had seen so many miracles. He then began sharing a story about a woman who came to their church with a huge mass in her colon. It was so large, he said, that you could see it moving beneath her skin. After he prayed over her, he said that she went into the bathroom and the mass came out and, when she returned, her dress was just hanging on her body because she had lost so much weight.

They had seen so many miracles but had not yet seen one in Glenda's health. As I continued talking to her, I boldly said, "Maybe you shouldn't have any more chemo. It is really making you sick. Instead, look to your Great Physician, God."

We exchanged contact information before I left and I followed up with her to see how she was doing. When I called, she was very sick and, in my heart, I don't know if she is still alive. I no longer have her contact info so I just pray for her anytime I think of her. I certainly hope and pray that she too received a miracle of healing from God.

The next day I was excited to share what had happened to me when Pastor Billy prayed for me. I told my friend Teresa and a few others who were nearby and this time I gave them the animated version. To give them a real sense of what had happened, I took my story to the next level and demonstrated the events of the evening. Teresa and everyone who was listening were so amazed that she said, "This could be a great ending of the book!" Everyone agreed. As I think back on her statement, realizing that the book is almost coming to a close, I pause. I don't want these last few pages to be thought of as an 'ending' but, rather instead, I want you to see it as a new, remarkable beginning!

This entire experience has led me to do more research on Christian healers. Let me be clear, I am not talking about metaphysical healers. I am talking about Christian men and women who are vessels that God uses to heal. All of this has opened my eyes to the world of the supernatural. I am constantly finding more and more fascinating information about God and healing.

My confidence and faith continue to increase daily. If you like to read or listen to CD's, I recommend Gloria Copeland's teachings on healing (www.kcm.org), Dodie Osteen's Healed Of Cancer and also Andrew Womack's wonderful teachings on healing (www.awmi.net)

Some of the scripture verses Dodie Osteen stood on during her battle with cancer can be located on this website, (http://hopefaithprayer.com/scriptures/healing-scriptures-dodie-osteen/).

My friendship with Teresa Tapp has continued to grow over the last couple of years. She invited me back to speak at another T-Tapp event that she was hosting. This time, I tried to perfect my speech and delivered what I thought was some great information to those who were in attendance.

During this particular trip, I decided it was time to visit my parents. It had been nine long years since I had seen my father. That's a very long time to go without seeing someone. Something spectacular happened during that visit. I realized that I had completely forgiven him after all these years. It was one of the happiest times of my life. I was able to enjoy spending the day with both of my parents without any anxiety. There was laughter and a peace that hovered over me the entire time. I realized a truly remarkable healing of my heart had also taken place.

I have to include in this chapter an incredible doctor I met at a conference - Dr. Rob Carlson! He taught me about the importance of keeping my hormones balanced and it has changed my life. He's actually a cardiologist who is also doing hormone work, specializing in the treatment of women. He really understands breast cancer and has done wonders in balancing my hormones. One of the things I like the most about him is that he takes the time to thoroughly explain everything to you and answers all of your questions. Thanks to him, I feel remarkable!

April 10th, 2011 *Well, can it get any better than this? Exactly two years have passed since I was first diagnosed.*

I am feeling the urge to plan a trip to San Jose. I love California and I would love to see my dear friend, Jan Skuba, whom I have known since I was fifteen. Plus, if you will remember from the first chapter, titled Good Friday, she is the one who put me in touch with the Eli. He and his wife were the ones who prayed for me over the phone right after I was diagnosed. I really want to see Jan and meet Eli and his wife in person.

I really enjoyed my visit. During my stay, I met Eli and we all made time to feed the homeless. After we finished working with those who were less fortunate than we are, a group of us went back to Eli's home and I met his wife, Judy. She had been healed from cancer after two years of trusting God and believing His word.

When she was first diagnosed, her cancer was very advanced. By the time she went to the doctor, it was so severe that blood was oozing from her breast and the cancer had metastasized to her brain. But, Judy put her trust in God and, by walking out her faith, God miraculously healed her.

While we were hanging out and discussing the topic of healing, Eli decides to pray for me. As he prayed, he spoke healing over my entire body. He prayed not only for me to be healed of cancer but also for the health of all of my organs, ligaments and my back – which had been hurting and felt like I had slipped a disc. Needless to say,

I was slain in the Spirit and it went right back into place.

It was a good thing that he asked me to stand by the sofa before he started praying. As I fell back, this awful sound came out of me, "Oof," and my friend Jan said, "Boo-ya!" For those of you who don't already know, Boo-ya is a slang term that is defined as an exclamation of joy, excitement or triumph. Thinking back on this, it makes me laugh. I really enjoyed that trip and it wasn't nearly as long as I wished it could have been.

In closing out this chapter, I can tell you with confidence that I know I am healed. I am staying on the path of healthy living and walking by faith each and every day. I am excited about life and look forward with joy and anticipation to the future that God has in store for me.

As I said earlier in the book, God had told me that one day I would share my story in order to take the fear out of the hearts of others. I knew that it was time to share the wealth of knowledge I had acquired on my journey.

Do you remember Lisa, the prayer partner who prayed for me at the church right after my diagnosis? Well, another amazing thing happened from my knowing her.

As I researched and talked to potential ghostwriters, I wasn't getting the response I was looking for. One day, God impressed upon my heart to ask her to help me. When I called her, she told me that when she was praying,

God told her to write. But, she didn't know what she was supposed to write. That was just two days prior to me calling her!

I tell her all the time that she 'gets me'! I find it amazing how God had connected us from the very beginning. Now, here we are at the beach compiling all of the details of my story, what a truly remarkable journey!

"This is the day that the Lord has made, I will rejoice and be glad in it."

Psalm 118:24

Thus says the Lord, "Stand in the ways and see, and ask for the old paths, where the good way is, and walk in it, then you will find rest for your souls."

Jeremiah 6:16

Laughter

We think of fun as a party, being outdoors, being with family, beach outings or a vacation with family. Webster's defines laughter as an inner quality, mood, or disposition and the sound or action that is produced. I, on the other hand, define it as a good medicine to the heart and soul.

If I can give you some advice, don't ever 'become' your disease. You can get so wrapped up in it that you stop living your life. I want to remind you that cancer is just visiting. If you have put your life on pause after being diagnosed, press the 'play' button and start living again. In fact, start living life large.

I am constantly reaching out to others that have been diagnosed, trying to share my insights and the things that I am learning along this journey. One day, I invited a woman over to my apartment who was diagnosed with breast cancer. She told me that she literally thought about her treatments every single minute of the day. I remember telling her, "You are not your disease." Immediately she said, "Yes, I am."

She had become so obsessed with the disease we call cancer that she was not living her life. Six months passed by and I ran into her one night when I was out. She asked what I had been doing and I told her that I had spent a fun evening at a wine bar with some of my friends. I asked her if she had been able to find anything fun to do herself.

She replied, "What's fun? I don't remember." She had forgotten how to enjoy her life. It could be as simple as reading a book, going to the movies, laughing with a friend or having a glass of wine.

I will admit that, in the beginning, it was hard to have fun. I remember trying to be perfect in all that I was doing. I recall putting great effort and constant thought into what I was eating or how much rest I was I getting. I also remember being careful to take all of my supplements and

174

seeking God through prayer, scripture reading and church.

For those who know me, moderation is not the first word that comes to mind. I have been told that I have a bigger than life personality. I have traveled all over, had lots of lovers, I've been married and I can party. But, I had to learn how to apply moderation in every area of my life in order to bring good health and well-being to my body, mind and spirit.

Laughter is more powerful than the most expensive or effective drugs! Did you know that those who laugh on a regular basis live longer, are healthier and make better decisions? Let's look at laughter and humor a little closer. If you haven't found a reason to laugh today, take a look in the mirror - that should help. We need to have a sense of humor and, if we can't laugh at ourselves, we leave the job to others. *"A cheerful mind works healing; a broken spirit dries up the bones." - Proverbs 17:22*

Every time we laugh it means we are getting healthier, stronger, younger, smarter, and blessings are flowing through our system. It's the best stress reliever. Laughter lowers blood pressure, helps you get a good night's sleep and it even increases your brain power. The best thing about laughter is it tears down walls and helps build relationships. In other words, it opens doors.

There is too much sadness in the world today. People are beaten down. Let them hear your laughter. There is healing in just hearing laughter. Let's be more like children. When we were children we knew how to laugh. Let's release the child in us. God has given us everything we need to keep us healthy and whole so dust off your laughing machine. It will stimulate your immune system and kick in what your body needs to heal and protect you from disease. *Jesus called a little child to Him, set him in the midst of them, and said, "Assuredly, I say to you, unless you are converted and become as little children, you will by no means enter the kingdom of heaven." – Matthew 18:2-3*

Negative emotions such as sadness, depression and anger slow the immune system way down and affect it in ways that we cannot see. When we laugh we release the healing power that God has placed inside of us. I've read of individuals who made sure that they only watched funny movies and stayed away from anything that brought out negative emotions like fear. They healed very quickly because they kept one of their best healing mechanisms turned on. *Job 8:21 – "God will fill your mouth with laughing and your lips with rejoicing."*

Those who laugh and have a good sense of humor and are easy to be around have more of the lovely NK cells that are known to kill cancer. I still love to hear or tell a good, clean joke or recount a funny past experience. It not only makes others laugh, but I also crack myself up. So, as it says in *Acts 20:24*

Then our mouths were filled with laughter and our tongues with singing. Then we said among the nations, "The Lord has done great things for us and we are glad. Psalm 126:2

If I Had to Do It All Over Again

As they say, hindsight is 20/20. I truly believe if I knew what I know now - and had consistently practiced these habits, I would not have had to live through the hell of a diagnosis of cancer.

If I had started - many years ago, truly forgiving and making sure there was no anger in my heart, all those cellular memories and the damage to my body would not have occurred. If I had been eating healthy by including the proper alkaline plant-based diet and live foods, then I may not be sitting her writing this book. If I had been exercising properly and balancing my hormones, I may have been one of the many who never get cancer.

But, living with a 'what if' mentality is not the way I want to be. In an odd kind of way, I am glad that I went through all of this now that I have the chance to look back. If I hadn't taken this journey, my life might not have changed for the better and I would have missed experiencing the true kindness of so many.

As I look back on all that I have learned, I am so grateful to really know, first-hand how the psalmist felt when he wrote,

"I will praise You, for I am fearfully and wonderfully made.[1] Marvelous are Your works, and that my soul knows very well." - Psalm 139:14

It is so true that God fearfully and wonderfully made each one of us in a way that our bodies can heal themselves from any disease. Knowledge of this truth is empowering! Knowing now what I have learned from researching and from my experiences, this book outlines a plan that I would make if I were diagnosed today.

The best part is, for those who are reading it, you can bypass all the time I invested in researching and all the time I wasted on fear. You can been spared the mental and physical effects that the fear of a diagnosis does to your body.

First and most importantly, get into agreement with God's promises for you and receive His healing. A powerful combination of God's grace and your faith will bring it

179

about. *"Be of good cheer, daughter, your faith has made you well." And she was made well from that hour.* – Jesus, in Matthew 9:22

Secondly, after being diagnosed, I would have rescheduled my clients for the next three weeks, found a place for my dog to stay and I would have checked myself into one of the following clinics that are known for getting you into the state of optimal health. They are, the Hippocrates Health Institute in Florida and The Optimal Health Institute (OHI) located in Texas and California. These are a few of the many alternative places to choose from. Be careful and prayerfully choose the best treatment methods. I give you these three because I feel they are reputable and will not take advantage of you.

One of the main purposes of getting away is to eliminate stress and calm yourself physically and emotionally. This will help you focus on detoxing, adjusting to dietary changes as well as getting your body into an alkaline state. It will also help you being away from the stress of your job and most importantly the fear of some of your family and friends. Another wonderful benefit of these places is that they prepare your food and juices as well as monitor your health and treat your needs accordingly.

By taking the step of going to a center like these, I believe you will save a lot of money in the long run. If I had been able to go to one of these places, I would have been able to get through some of the detox process much sooner. I would have also gotten my body into an alkaline state long before I did. The key information I would have received from these experts would have also allowed me to relax a lot sooner.

After going to one of these centers, I would then return home and find a good, highly recommended local naturopathic doctor to work with in case I needed additional advice and/or treatments.

Knowing what I know now, I believe the journey would have been much shorter in receiving my healing and clean bill of health. But, I would have missed some of the interesting situations I experienced along my journey.

I recommend highly that you purchase a Vita Mix and a juicer and set up your kitchen for your new healthier way of living. I'm still doing this because I now know my body can heal itself from any past damage and that it will help me to remain healthy and cancer free. *"Affliction will not rise up a second time."* - Nahum 1:9

If you will take the time and do your homework, you will find that there is a lot of amazing information out there about the natural cures for cancer. Once again, approach your search with prayer because there is a lot of mis-information out there.

If your healing isn't manifested immediately, keep walking

in blind faith. Choose a protocol and stick to it, allowing time to see the results and time for your body to heal. It's up to you to take responsibility for your body. *"Do you not know that your body is the temple of the Holy Spirit who is in you, whom you have from God, and that you are not your own? For you were bought at a price; therefore glorify God in your body and in your spirit, which are God's" – 1st Corinthians 6:19*

When you get your clean bill of health, don't get lazy, stay with this new lifestyle and live a long healthy life in the name of Jesus. My hope and prayer for you is for you to realize that God has designed a miracle for you. Just ask for it, it has your name on it. Your miracle is right around the corner. Just claim it! *"Ask, and it will be given to you; seek, and you will find; knock, and it will be opened to you. For everyone who asks receives, and those who seek find, and to one who knocks it will be opened." - Jesus, in Matthew 7:7-8*

"Those who wait on the Lord
Shall renew their strength;
They shall mount up with wings like eagles,
They shall run and not be weary,
They shall walk and not faint."
Isaiah 40:31

Memorial to Iggy

Saying goodbye is never easy!

For all of you pet lovers out there, you know what it means to lose a member of your family. It tears your heart right out of your chest.

I rescued Iggy when he was five years old and his life started out hard. When I got him he had heart worms and his joints - especially his hips, were not in the best condition. So the beginning of our time together was me taking care of him, making sure he finished the heart worm treatments, teaching him things like how walk on a leash like a gentleman and the rules of my home.

One rule for instance, was "You cannot pull a plate of Thanksgiving turkey off the counter and run around the house with a piece of turkey in your mouth". My friend Victor and his kids will always remember that incident. To them it's still hilarious. Iggy was so smart and eager to please and he never did that again!

As our time together went on, he would always be there to give comfort and watch over me. When I was diagnosed with breast cancer, he went through all my ups and downs with me, always by my side from diagnosis to my healing.

But I didn't get Iggy as a pup and he was now showing signs of getting older. The worst was going blind, I knew he was losing his sight but didn't know how bad until one early morning he walked off a three foot wall and injured his right leg. I felt like the worst mom in the world, just days before he could go right up to the same wall and jump down, to play with the little dog from next door.

Now it was my time again to be by his side and protect him from things he could not see and to keep his stress as low as possible. For a dog, especially a working dog (Iggy was a Blue Heeler), bred to herd sheep and cattle; losing their eyesight is a very hard adjustment.

In October of 2013 I moved us out of our home, which Iggy was accustomed, and into a new place for a little over a year. In February of 2015 I packed us up and we took a road trip and stayed out on ten acres for me to rest and recuperate from a long six months. Everything was going great until one day I didn't get to my Iggy fast enough and he fell off some old wooden stairs into a hole and injured the same right leg.

The worst part of the accident was the fall scared him so badly he was traumatized and went into shock. Once again I didn't get to him fast enough and he got injured. I still beat myself up over this, his screams still play in my head if I let them.

I nursed him and thought he was getting better, but within 24 hours he went downhill fast, I knew he was tired and losing his will to live. Now was the time to pack up the car and get him back to Austin, I knew what had to be done and I wanted him with his Vet Rebecca Davies, because they know each other and she is such a kind and compassionate woman.

Getting him to the car was very tricky because he

had lost his ability to walk; my big strong dog was now unable to walk and was frightened and hurting. I got him to the car as best I could but I know I hurt him and for that I am so sorry. The whole three hours back to Austin I kept telling him how much I loved him, what an amazing dog he was, but most importantly I kept thanking him for picking me as his mom.

Once we got to the vets office it was as if he was saying I'm so ready I could never make the trip to Florida and it was OK now to say "Goodbye"

It was a very peaceful ending. I know I made the right decision, it's one all pet owners have to make sooner or later it seems. It is the hardest and most loving decision you can make; to not let a beautiful creature of God suffer anymore.

I want to thank Rebecca Davies and the staff at Arbor animal hospital for their gentle touch and kindness they always showed my beloved Iggy.

Iggy you will forever be my soul dog and we will see each other again!

In memory of Iggy

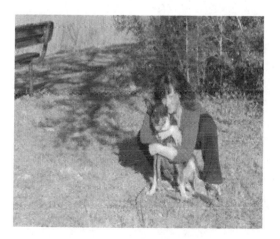

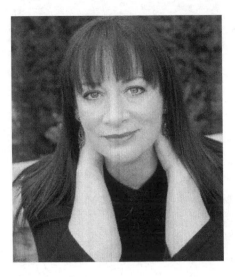

Thank you so much for reading about my adventures. It has been almost seven years since my diagnosis of breast cancer and I am alive and well! I am out and about doing what I am passionate about; speaking at all kinds of events and venues on the importance of "Prevention" and telling my story with all kinds of fun and enlightening information. Yes you can live a long life after a diagnosis of cancer.

I would love for you to be there for many more of my adventures, please head on over to my website www.VenusDeMarco.org and sign up for my newsletter.

If you need a speaker for an event, please reach out to me.

To your health and long life!

Venus

34296536R00116

Made in the USA
San Bernardino, CA
24 May 2016